Intracranial Stereotactic Radiosurgery

Editor

BRUCE E. POLLOCK

NEUROSURGERY
CLINICS OF NORTH AMERICA

www.neurosurgery.theclinics.com

October 2013 • Volume 24 • Number 4

ELSEVIER

1600 John F. Kennedy Boulevard • Suite 1800 • Philadelphia, Pennsylvania, 19103-2899

http://www.theclinics.com

NEUROSURGERY CLINICS OF NORTH AMERICA Volume 24, Number 4
October 2013 ISSN 1042-3680, ISBN-13: 978-0-323-22727-8

Editor: Jessica McCool

Neurosurgery Clinics of North America (ISSN 1042-3680) is published quarterly by Elsevier Inc., 360 Park Avenue South, New York, NY 10010-1710. Months of issue are January, April, July, and October. Business and Editorial Offices: 1600 John F. Kennedy Blvd., Suite 1800, Philadelphia, PA 19103-2899. Customer Service Office: 11830 Westline Industrial Drive, St. Louis, MO 63146. Periodicals postage paid at New York, NY, and additional mailing offices. Subscription prices are $360.00 per year (US individuals), $552.00 per year (US institutions), $393.00 per year (Canadian individuals), $674.00 per year (Canadian institutions), $502.00 per year (international individuals), $674.00 per year (international institutions), $177.00 per year (US students), and $243.00 per year (international students). International air speed delivery is included in all *Clinics* subscription prices. All prices are subject to change without notice. **POSTMASTER:** Send address changes to *Neurosurgery Clinics of North America*, Elsevier Periodicals Customer Service, 11830 Westline Industrial Drive, St. Louis, MO 63146. **Customer Service: 1-800-654-2452 (US and Canada). From outside the US and Canada, call: 1-314-453-7041. Fax: 1-314-453-5170. E-mail: JournalsCustomerService-usa@elsevier.com (for print support) and journalsonlinesupport-usa@elsevier.com (for online support).**

Reprints. For copies of 100 or more, of articles in this publication, please contact the Commercial Reprints Department, Elsevier Inc., 360 Park Avenue South, New York, NY 10010-1710. Tel. (212) 633-3874; Fax: (212) 633-3820; E-mail: reprints@elsevier.com.

Neurosurgery Clinics of North America is covered in *MEDLINE/PubMed (Index Medicus), EMBASE/Excerpta Medica,* and *Current Contents/Clinical Medicine (CC/CM).*

Printed and bound by CPI Group (UK) Ltd, Croydon, CR0 4YY

Transferred to digital print 2012

Contributors

EDITOR

BRUCE E. POLLOCK, MD
Professor of Neurosurgery, Departments of
Neurological Surgery and Radiation Oncology,
Mayo Clinic College of Medicine, Rochester,
Minnesota

AUTHORS

ROMAIN CARRON, MD
Department of Stereotactic and Functional
Neurosurgery, Gammaknife Unit, La Timone
University Hospital, Marseille, France

MICHAEL D. CHAN, MD
Department of Radiation Oncology, Wake
Forest School of Medicine, Winston-Salem,
North Carolina

STEVEN D. CHANG, MD
Professor, Department of Neurosurgery,
Robert C. and Jeannette Powell Professor in
the Neurosciences, Stanford University,
Stanford, California

ANTONIO A.F. DE SALLES, MD, PhD
Head of Stereotactic Surgery Section,
Professor of Neurosurgery, Departments of
Neurosurgery and Radiation Oncology, David
Geffen School of Medicine, University of
California Los Angeles, Los Angeles, California;
Chief, HCor Neuroscience, Sao Paulo, Brazil

CHRISTINE DELSANTI, MD
Department of Stereotactic and Functional
Neurosurgery, Gammaknife Unit, La Timone
University Hospital, Marseille, France

JOHN C. FLICKINGER, MD, FACR
Department of Radiation Oncology, University
of Pittsburgh Medical Center, Pittsburgh,
Pennsylvania

WILLIAM A. FRIEDMAN, MD
Professor and Chairman, Department of
Neurologic Surgery, University of Florida,
Gainesville, Florida

ALESSANDRA A. GORGULHO, MD, MSc
Adjunct Assistant Professor, Departments of
Neurosurgery and Radiation Oncology, David
Geffen School of Medicine, University of
California Los Angeles, Los Angeles, California;
Clinical Scientific Chief, HCor Neuroscience,
Sao Paulo, Brazil

SHUNYA HANAKITA, MD
Department of Neurosurgery, The University of
Tokyo Hospital, Bunkyo-ku, Tokyo, Japan

TOSHINORI HASEGAWA MD
Department of Neurosurgery, Gamma Knife
Center, Komaki City Hospital, Komaki, Aichi
Prefecture, Japan

YOSHINORI HIGUCHI, MD, PhD
Department of Neurological Surgery, Chiba
University Graduate School of Medicine,
Chiba, Japan

JANA JEŽKOVÁ, MD, PhD
Third Department of Internal Medicine, First
Faculty of Medicine, Charles University,
Prague, Czech Republic

HIDEYUKI KANO, MD, PhD
Research Assistant Professor, Department
of Neurological Surgery, The Center for
Image-Guided Neurosurgery, UPMC
Presbyterian, University of Pittsburgh School
of Medicine, Pittsburgh, Pennsylvania

SYED AFTAB KARIM, MD
Department of Neurosurgery, Stanford
University School of Medicine, Stanford,
California

ANDRAS A. KEMENY, FRCS, MD
National Centre for Stereotactic Radiosurgery, Royal Hallamshire Hospital, Sheffield, South Yorkshire, United Kingdom

TOMOYUKI KOGA, MD, PhD
Department of Neurosurgery, The University of Tokyo Hospital, Bunkyo-ku, Tokyo, Japan

DOUGLAS KONDZIOLKA, MD, MSc, FRCSC, FACS
Professor of Neurosurgery and Radiation Oncology; Vice-Chair, Clinical Research Director, Center for Advanced Radiosurgery, NYU Langone Medical Center, New York University, New York, New York

GIUSEPPE LANZINO, MD
Professor, Department of Neurologic Surgery, Mayo Clinic, Rochester, Minnesota

MICHAEL J. LINK, MD
Department of Neurological Surgery, Mayo Clinic College of Medicine, Rochester, Minnesota

ROMAN LIŠČÁK, MD, PhD
Associate Professor, Stereotactic and Radiation Neurosurgery, Na Homolce Hospital, Prague, Czech Republic

L. DADE LUNSFORD, MD, FACS
Lars Leksell Professor and Distinguished Professor, The Center for Image-Guided Neurosurgery, Department of Neurological Surgery, University of Pittsburgh Medical Center, Pittsburgh, Pennsylvania

JOSEF MAREK, MD, DrSc
Professor, Third Department of Internal Medicine, First Faculty of Medicine, Charles University, Prague, Czech Republic

NANCY MCLAUGHLIN, MD
Assistant Professor, Departments of Neurosurgery and Radiation Oncology, David Geffen School of Medicine, University of California Los Angeles, Los Angeles, California

AKITAKE MUKASA, MD, PhD
Department of Neurosurgery, The University of Tokyo Hospital, Bunkyo-ku, Tokyo, Japan

XAVIER MURRACCIOLE, MD
Professor, Aix-Marseille University; Department of Radiation Oncology, La Timone University Hospital, Marseille, France

OSAMU NAGANO, MD, PhD
Gamma Knife House, Chiba Cardiovascular Center, Ichihara, Japan

GÁBOR NAGY, MD, PhD
Department of Neuro-Oncology, National Institute of Neurosciences, Budapest, Hungary

JULIO L.B. PEREIRA, MD
Fellow, Stereotactic Surgery, Departments of Neurosurgery and Radiation Oncology, David Geffen School of Medicine, University of California Los Angeles, Los Angeles, California

BRUCE E. POLLOCK, MD
Professor of Neurosurgery, Departments of Neurological Surgery and Radiation Oncology, Mayo Clinic College of Medicine, Rochester, Minnesota

DENIS PORCHERON, PhD
Professor, Department of Stereotactic and Functional Neurosurgery, Gammaknife Unit; Department of Radiation Oncology, La Timone University Hospital, Marseille, France

JEAN RÉGIS, MD
Professor, Aix-Marseille University; Department of Stereotactic and Functional Neurosurgery, Gammaknife Unit, La Timone University Hospital, Marseille, France

PIERRE-HUGUES ROCHE, MD
Professor, Aix-Marseille University; Department of Neurosurgery, Northern University Hospital, Marseille, France

KUNIAKI SAITO, MD
Department of Neurosurgery, The University of Tokyo Hospital, Bunkyo-ku, Tokyo, Japan

NOBUHITO SAITO, MD, PhD
Department of Neurosurgery, The University of Tokyo Hospital, Bunkyo-ku, Tokyo, Japan

TORU SERIZAWA, MD, PhD
Tokyo Gamma Unit Center, Tsukiji Neurologic Clinic, Tokyo, Japan

EDWARD G. SHAW, MD, MA
Department of Radiation Oncology, Wake Forest School of Medicine, Winston-Salem, North Carolina

JASON P. SHEEHAN, MD, PhD
Professor, Department of Neurological Surgery, University of Virginia, Charlottesville, Virginia

MASAHIRO SHIN, MD, PhD
Department of Neurosurgery, The University of Tokyo Hospital, Bunkyo-ku, Tokyo, Japan

SCOTT L. STAFFORD, MD
Department of Radiation Oncology, Mayo Clinic College of Medicine, Rochester, Minnesota

SHOTA TANAKA, MD
Department of Neurosurgery, The University of Tokyo Hospital, Bunkyo-ku, Tokyo, Japan

STEPHEN B. TATTER, MD, PhD
Department of Neurosurgery, Wake Forest School of Medicine, Winston-Salem, North Carolina

JEAN-MARC THOMASSIN, MD
Professor, Aix-Marseille University; Department of ENT, Head and Neck Surgery, La Timone University Hospital, Marseille, France

CHUN-PO YEN, MD
Resident Physician, Department of Neurological Surgery, University of Virginia, Charlottesville, Virginia

JACKY T. YEUNG, MD
Department of Neurosurgery, Yale University School of Medicine, New Haven, Connecticut

Contents

removal followed by radiosurgery to the residual tumor is proposed. The authors' cohort is unique with respect to the size of the population and the length of the follow-up, and demonstrates the efficacy and safety of VS radiosurgery, with particular regard to its high rate of hearing preservation.

This article summarizes tumor control and functional outcomes of stereotactic radiosurgery (SRS) for patients with nonvestibular schwannomas, in comparison with those treated with microsurgical resection. To date, surgical resection has been a common treatment for nonvestibular schwannomas. Because these tumors are generally benign, complete tumor resection is a desirable curative treatment. However, it is almost infeasible to completely remove these tumors without any complications, even for experienced neurosurgeons, because of adherence to surrounding critical structures such as cranial nerves, brainstem, or vessels. SRS provides a good tumor control rate with much less morbidity than microsurgical resection.

Multi-session stereotactic radiosurgery (SRS) enables a high dose per fraction to be delivered to the tumor bed with rapid dose falloff that allows for sparing of critical structures, resulting in less radiation-associated toxicity. In this article, the authors review the basic concepts and techniques of multi-session SRS, indications for this technique, outcomes from single-session and multi-session SRS using 3 commonly treated benign intracranial tumors (meningiomas, vestibular schwannomas, pituitary adenomas), and discuss why multi-session SRS is an attractive approach for the treatment of these tumors.

Chordomas and chondrosarcomas are rare, slow-growing, locally aggressive tumors with high recurrence rates. Stereotactic radiosurgery (SRS) is an important management option for patients with recurrent or residual chordomas and chondrosarcomas. Glomus jugulare tumor are rare highly vascularized tumors that arise from the paraganglionic structures of the glossopharyngeal and vagal nerves. Because of their highly vascular nature and surgically formidable anatomic location, curative resection often proves challenging. SRS can be used as an up-front treatment or as an additional treatment for patients with recurrent or residual glomus jugulare tumor after surgical resection.

Stereotactic radiosurgery for intracranial arteriovenous malformations (AVMs) has been performed since the 1970s. When an AVM is treated with radiosurgery, radiation injury to the vascular endothelium induces the proliferation of smooth muscle cells and the elaboration of extracellular collagen, which leads to progressive stenosis and obliteration of the AVM nidus. Obliteration after AVM radiosurgery ranges from 60% to 80%, and relates to the size of the AVM and the prescribed radiation dose. The major drawback of radiosurgical AVM treatment is the risk of bleeding during the latent period (typically 2 years) between treatment and AVM thrombosis.

NEUROSURGERY CLINICS OF NORTH AMERICA

NEUROSURGERY CLINICS OF NORTH AMERICA

FORTHCOMING ISSUES

January 2014
Advances in Neuromodulation
Won Kim, MD, Antonio De Salles, MD,
and Nader Pouratian, MD, Editors

April 2014
Minimally Invasive Spine Surgery
Richard Fessler, MD and Zachary Smith, MD,
Editors

July 2014
Endovascular Management of
Cerebrovascular Disease
Ricardo Hanel, MD, Ciaran Powers, MD, and
Eric Sauvageau, MD, Editors

RECENT ISSUES

July 2013
Neurocritical Care in Neurosurgery
Paul A. Nyquist, MD, Marek A. Mirski, MD,
and Rafael J. Tamargo, MD, Editor

April 2013
Spinal Deformity Surgery
Christopher P. Ames, MD, Brian Jian, MD, and
Christopher I. Shaffrey, MD, Editors

January 2013
Malignant Tumors of the Skull Base
Orin Bloch, MD and Franco DeMonte, MD,
FRCSC, FACS Editors

RELATED INTEREST

Surgical Oncology Clinics of North America, July 2013 (Vol. 22, Issue 3),
Practical Radiation Oncology for Surgeons
Christopher G. Willett, MD, Editor
http://www.surgonc.theclinics.com/

Preface
Intracranial Stereotactic Radiosurgery

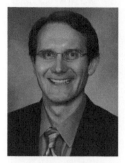

Bruce E. Pollock, MD
Editor

The practice of medicine is marked by transformative changes that push forward its science in the hope of improving patient outcomes. Over the past 60 years, stereotactic radiosurgery (SRS) has evolved from a concept, to an investigatory procedure, before becoming an accepted treatment option for benign or malignant tumors, vascular malformations, and functional disorders. Furthermore, SRS has grown from a single-fraction technique for intracranial pathologic abnormalities to now include multisession SRS and extracranial indications. Radiosurgery is now a mandatory component of postgraduate education for both neurologic surgeons and radiation oncologists. Without exaggeration, SRS should be considered one of the most significant advances in these fields over the past half-century.

The goal of this issue of *Neurosurgery Clinics of North America* is to provide a succinct but complete review of contemporary intracranial SRS. The authors of each article are recognized for their expertise and include neurosurgeons and radiation oncologists from around the world. Each article is clinically focused and devoted to a single topic or pathologic condition. It is hoped that this issue will be worthwhile not only for neurologic surgeons and radiation oncologists but also for a wide range of physicians and physicians-in-training across multiple disciplines who care for patients with neurologic diseases.

Bruce E. Pollock, MD
Departments of Neurological Surgery and
Radiation Oncology
Mayo Clinic College of Medicine
200 1st SW Streeet
Rochester, MN 55905, USA

E-mail address:
Pollock.Bruce@mayo.edu

http://dx.doi.org/10.1016/j.nec.2013.06.004
1042-3680/13/$ – see front matter © 2013 Published by Elsevier Inc.

neurosurgery.theclinics.com

Intracranial Stereotactic Radiosurgery
Concepts and Techniques

Antonio A.F. De Salles, MD, PhD[a,b,*],
Alessandra A. Gorgulho, MD, MSc[a,b],
Julio L.B. Pereira, MD[a,b], Nancy McLaughlin, MD[a,b]

KEYWORDS

- Stereotactic radiosurgery • Gamma Knife • Linear accelerator • Novalis • Cyberknife
- Tomotherapy

KEY POINTS

Readers of this article will learn:

- The history of device development for radiosurgery.
- The technical nuances of each intracranial radiosurgery device.
- Step-by-step performance of a radiosurgery procedure.
- The need of a team approach in radiosurgery.
- The expansion of intracranial radiosurgery to other areas of the body.

INTRODUCTION

Stereotactic radiosurgery evolved based on two good ideas. First, treating a lesion in human tissues with external beam radiation, described by Kohl 18 years after the discovery of X-rays.[1] The second hinged on the work of Horsley and Clarke, neurosurgeon and mathematician, respectively, who developed a tool to localize intracranial structures in three dimensions. This work resulted in a stereotactic atlas of the primate brain published in 1908. An atlas that combined the use of this development was the subject of Spiegel's reported human stereotactic atlas in 1952.[2,3]

The concept of applying focal X-rays as a therapeutic tool evolved using spiral converging beams, pendulum-directed beams, and finally rigid hemispheric distributed beams directed with stereotactic precision.[4] It was Lars Leksell, a practicing functional neurosurgeon at Karolinska University in Stockholm, Sweden, who integrated stereotactic precision with the penetrating capability and the tissue effect of the photon beam. As widely described, Leksell attached an X-ray tube to his stereotactic arc centered frame and delivered radiosurgery to the first patient submitted to the technique, targeting the trigeminal ganglion for treatment of trigeminal neuralgia. The term "radiosurgery" was coined.[2]

Radiosurgery evolved during the last half of the twentieth century linked to the explosion of imaging techniques.[5] Because it was dependent on ventriculography, cysternography, and angiography, the applications of radiosurgery were largely limited to pathologies visualized by these techniques. Functional applications were based on principles of functional neurosurgery localization, for example using the anterior commissure and

Disclosures: The authors have nothing to disclose.
a Department of Neurosurgery, David Geffen School of Medicine, University of California Los Angeles, Los Angeles, CA 90095, USA; b Department of Radiation Oncology, David Geffen School of Medicine, University of California Los Angeles, Los Angeles, CA 90095, USA
* Corresponding author. Department of Neurosurgery, David Geffen School of Medicine, University of California Los Angeles, 10495 Le Conte Avenue, Suite 2120, Los Angeles, CA 90095.
E-mail addresses: afdesalles@yahoo.com; adesalles@mednet.ucla.edu

Neurosurg Clin N Am 24 (2013) 491–498
http://dx.doi.org/10.1016/j.nec.2013.07.001
1042-3680/13/$ – see front matter © 2013 Elsevier Inc. All rights reserved.

posterior commissure seen by ventriculography to guide targeting. Meckel cave contrast material injection and cysternography provided visualization of targets, such as the trigeminal ganglion in the Meckel's cave and the acoustic neuroma's prominence in the cerebellopontine angle, previously not seen in plain skull radiographs.[6] Angiography provided the visualization of arteriovenous malformations (AVMs), making them the classic application of radiosurgery starting in 1972.[7] The buildup of radiosurgery applications with the introduction of structural diseases, such as acoustic neuromas and AVMs, increased the demand for affordable radiosurgery throughout the world. During the early 1980s there were less than 10 radiosurgery devices serving the world's population: three Gamma Knives and a few proton facilities.

Modern neurosurgery develops toward minimally invasive procedures, therefore radiosurgery has gained space. The multidisciplinary nature of the procedure involving the neurosurgeon, radiation oncologist, and medical physicist aims to minimize the risks and to improve the treatment success rate. This has been met with great acceptance by patients and payers alike. Radiosurgery has an important therapeutic role in the management of brain tumors, AVMs, and trigeminal neuralgia, and continues to expand its applications, including selected functional disorders of the brain, such as epilepsy.[8,9]

The success of intracranial radiosurgery has also spread to the spine and other areas of the body,[10] revolutionizing the practice of radiation oncology. The same impact of radiosurgery in general neurosurgery is being repeated in other surgical specialties, such as thoracic surgery.[11] The clinical importance of radiosurgery expedited the development of new technologies capable of increased speed, comfort, and effects of radiosurgery for its diverse applications.

Today there are four major photon energy radiosurgery devices competing in the market based on advantages and disadvantages of respective intended specific applications and strategies of planning the treatment (**Table 1**). Regardless of the approach, the fundamental concepts of radiosurgery include high doses of radiation, minimal doses in surrounding structures, stereotactic localization, use of computerized dosimetry planning, and a highly accurate radiation delivery system.[12–14]

BASIC CONCEPTS
Ionizing Radiation

Ionizing radiation for radiosurgery is any radiant entity that has enough energy to remove an electron from an atom, thus creating ions, which interact with the living tissue in the target generating a biologic response. Gamma rays are

---

Table 1
Summary of the capabilities of each technique routinely used for stereotactic radiosurgery and stereotactic radiotherapy planning

Modality	Indications	Key Features	Limitations
Circular collimator (single)	Small round targets, functional radiosurgery applications	Fast delivery, usually homogeneous (if diameter $\geq$10 mm)	Limited to small and round targets, rapid planning
Multiple isocenters	Small-to-medium irregularly shaped target	Conformal, inhomogeneous	Slow delivery, inhomogeneous, time-consuming planning
Dynamic-shaped beam	Small-to-medium irregularly shaped target	Conformal, homogeneous, fast radiation delivery	Loose conformality with large targets because of beam overlap
Static-shaped beam	Large irregularly shaped target	Conformal, homogeneous, fast radiation delivery	More dose through the path of the beam, usually time-consuming planning
Pencil beam painting	Irregularly shaped target	Conformal, homogeneous	Slow radiation delivery
Intensity modulation	Large irregularly shaped target	Conformal, tighter dose distribution, better sparing of organ at risk	Slow radiation delivery, usually inhomogeneous, strict delivery quality control

ionizing radiation originating from an excited nucleus of cobalt 60. This nucleus continuously gets rid of excess energy by emitting electromagnetic radiation, known as gamma ray. X-rays, however, are generated when an energized electron hits a heavy weight metal and looses energy in the form of a photon. This electromagnetic species has the same biologic effect on the targeted living tissue as a gamma ray. These photon beans generate free radicals that interact with molecules of DNA causing cell death, cell inability to divide, or modification of cell function. Radiosurgery takes advantage of the linear propagation of electromagnetic energy and its ability to interact with living matter to provoke the intended therapeutic reaction in the target tissue.

Another important factor of ionizing radiation for radiosurgery is the particulate energy. Because of the unique capability to stop its propagation at the point of maximal energy delivery in the tissue, a phenomenon called Bragg peak, it is very attractive for radiosurgery. It spares the tissue beyond the target, contrary to photons that irradiate beyond the target site. Particulate energies are produced in large cyclotrons where electrons are spanned out of the outer atomic layer and the nuclei are directed to the intended target by powerful magnets. In the case of protons, the hydrogen ion is the one spanned in the cyclotron. Historically, protons and alpha particles prominent of spanned helium beams established radiosurgery for pituitary tumors and had a major impact in the treatment of AVMs.[15,16] Because of its at least 30 times order of magnitude price compared with photon-based techniques, the particulate energy was used in only a few academic centers worldwide.[16] Modern particle accelerators dedicated to medical purpose are starting to become available. However, the price is still at least of 10 orders of magnitude of the current available dedicated radiosurgery system on the market.[17]

Radiosurgery Procedure

Understanding all of the steps of the radiosurgery procedure is essential to optimize results and reduce risks. Regardless of the method of delivery, it is important to follow all the safety steps of the procedure, because there is no equipment that is human error proof. Moreover, radiosurgery is prone to repetitive error. Because the effects of the treatment are not immediately seen, a large number of patients can be treated based on a single human error.[18] Radiosurgery should not be performed without a very well trained team made up of radiation technologists, medical physicists, radiation oncologists, and neurosurgeons.

The first step is a daily quality assurance routine to check basic aspects of the delivery system and software, and the precision of the delivery device. This should be followed by correct application of the stereotactic guiding device, either frameless or with a frame. A routine protocol of treatment delivery followed harmonically by all team members is essential.

The preparation for the procedure is based on acquisition of exquisite quality imaging dictated by the pathology. Integration of all imaging modalities, such as computed tomography (CT), CT angiography, magnetic resonance imaging, magnetic resonance angiography, conventional angiogram, and positron emission tomography, is desirable in modern radiosurgery systems. The treatment plan consists of a careful analysis of the image quality and the fusion of all images available to be registered in the same stereotactic space. The target volume is defined based on the composite of information of all images. The best dose distribution to affect the target and spare normal structures surrounding the disease is the goal of radiosurgery treatment, requiring the expertise of the physicist, the radiation oncologist, and the neurosurgeon. Each one brings to the radiosurgery plan the understanding of dose deposition, dose effect, and anatomic pitfalls known by each specialty. All specialists evaluate the isodose distribution, the dose volume histogram, the conformity index, and the feasibility of the radiosurgery system to delivery reliably and in an acceptable time frame the treatment plan.[5,8,9]

Radiosurgery Team

Radiosurgery is based on a multidisciplinary concept. The physicist brings knowledge of the device, the neurosurgeon of the anatomy, and the radiation oncologist of the interaction of ionizing radiation with living tissue. This concept generated a novel specialty overlap but none of the domains is able to independently perform the procedure within safe and optimized standards. In the operating room the neurosurgeon needs the anesthesiologist, the specialized nurse, the technicians, the electrophysiologist, and so on. Similarly, in radiosurgery the multiple professionals are necessary. This concept has been met with resistance in certain institutions, mainly related to the ego driven in each specialty and the economic interests of each specialist. This has led to major complications, harm to patients, and degradation of the method. Because the development of a field hinges on a well-established base of knowledge, radiosurgery only progresses when the basics of physics, radiobiology, anatomy, and clinical skills are well established. This occurs only with the participation of professionals working and dedicated to each of these fields of knowledge. Although economic pressure leads certain institutions to abolish or ostracize one of the components of the team, the consequences are lack of progress, increased risks for the patients, and poor results. The harmonic work of the radiosurgery team has provided for a minimally invasive approach, better quality of life for patients, and novel therapies for yet untreatable diseases.[8,19] Radiosurgery has taken a position of being responsible for 15% to 30% of the neurosurgery cases in major departments of neurosurgery.[20]

DEVICES FOR RADIOSURGERY
Gamma Knife

Leksell, searching for the best approach to perform his radiosurgery, evolved from an X-ray tube attached to his stereotactic device to the proton beam crossfire technique in Upsalla, Sweden, and finally settling with cobalt-60 photon beam as the most practical energy to have a hospital-based radiosurgery device. The Gamma Knife idea was born.[18] It was designed to be a turn-on turnkey device with minimal dependence on technical aspects that would hinder the neurosurgeon's interest in radiosurgery. Although the Gamma Knife is simple and designed for practicality, initially only stereotactic surgeons saw the reach of the device in neurosurgery. Today, even general neurosurgeons are using the Leksell Gamma Knife (Elekta AB, Stockholm, Sweden). Contemporary with Leksell's effort to develop a practical radiosurgery device, a patient in London was treated with a linear accelerator (Linac) for the first time in 1953,[21] leading to the development of the modern Linac. The first Gamma Knife was inaugurated in 1969, spreading around the world as the instrument of choice for radiosurgery.

The Leksell Gamma Knife, developed for brain radiosurgery, is currently used worldwide and is considered the gold standard for radiosurgery quality and precision. The system consists of simultaneous delivery of gamma rays generated by cobalt-60 sources directed to a single focus, machined to better than 0.3-mm precision. The precision of the Gamma Knife procedure depends, however, on imaging quality, appropriate stereotactic device fixation, quality of the planning, and strategic use of single or multiple isocenters to achieve the best possible conformity of the radiation volume to the volume of the lesion being treated. This requires experience of the user, although the planning optimization algorithm currently available in the planning software (Gamma Plan, Elekta AB) provides for possible standardization of the radiosurgery planning procedure. Although algorithms can never substitute for medical expertise, this can be a valuable tool for radiosurgeons still building up their expertise.

LGK Perfexion (Elekta AB) is the latest generation Gamma Knife containing 192 cobalt-60 sources arranged in conical configuration (**Fig. 1**). It is possible to combine the use of different beam sizes (4, 8, and 16 mm) with single or multiple isocenters to generate complex conformal plans adjusted to the shape of the lesion. It is possible to treat cervical spine lesions until vertebrae C3. It also has a noninvasive frame with a mouth block, which allows for short fractionated schemes to be performed. Despite this recent feature, the bulk of the experience with the Gamma Knife was built up with single doses.[9]

Gamma Knife units deliver gamma ray (cobalt 60) with a half-life of roughly 5 years. The output is more than 3.5 Gy per minute when the source is new. It has only circular collimators; therefore, multiple isocenters are necessary for irregular-shaped lesions. The positioning of the patient is based on stereotactic frame and it is dedicated to intracranial and possibly high cervical lesions. The important disadvantages of the system are the need of reloading the cobalt-60 source within 5 to 10 years, the need of an invasive fixation device, and the limitation of reaching only to C3 level.[13]

Linac-Based Systems

Linac radiosurgery systems generate a single high-energy X-ray beam that is focus by special

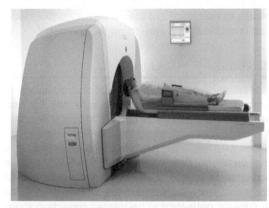

Fig. 1. Gamma Knife Perfexion featuring a robotic table and the automatic exchange of collimator size for multiple isocenters to allow complete robotic conduction of the radiosurgery treatment. (*Courtesy of* Elekta, Crawley, United Kingdom; with permission.)

collimators, either cone or multileaf, with the intent to narrow, modulate, or shape the beam to the tumor volume. It was developed starting in the 1980s to popularize radiosurgery to all hospitals capable of treating cancer patients with conventional radiation therapy. Although developed since the 1950s for large fields of radiation using fractionated schemes and capable of effectively treating cancer throughout the body, the Linac was not designed to deliver radiation with the precision required for radiosurgery. Therefore, adaptation of this machine to be as precise as the Gamma Knife unit allowed popularization of the radiosurgery technique.[22] The Linac now is the most frequently used device for delivery of radiosurgery in the world.

By 2006, more than 40 million patients with cancer had already been treated with Linac technology. Only 30 years after the initial use of the Linac in oncology, with complete establishment of the technology, was the first Linac-based radiosurgery treatment implemented. In the meantime, proof of concept of radiosurgery was also accomplished with the proton beam, including a dosimetric approach to single-dose radiation[23] and other approaches with rotation of cobalt-60 sources.[24] Finally, an Argentinean neurosurgeon saw the versatility and cost-effectiveness of the Linac, adapting it to radiosurgery. While working in France, Betty and Derechinsky[25] aligned the head of a patient in different angles in relation to the beam line of a Linac to treat an AVM. They gained a place in history as the first physicians to perform radiosurgery using the Linac approach. Their idea was promptly followed in Italy,[26] Germany,[27] and the United States.[28,29] These three reports set the stage for the development of the most accepted and versatile approach to perform radiosurgery today, and for the development of such approaches as the Cyberknife and the TomoTherapy High-Art system. Winston and Lutz[29] working in Boston adapted their Linac and developed the methodic steps of quality assurance and precision radiosurgery using the Linac. The Linac approach was initially heavily criticized because of imprecision of the machine in its rotational axis, mostly by Gamma Knife users who had established that technique as the gold standard of precision in the field. Criticism persisted until the development of a dedicated Linac for radiosurgery as a commercial product, the Novalis system (Brainlab, Feldkirchen, Germany).[30]

The Novalis system is an integrated system featuring treatment planning and treatment delivery for intracranial pathologies and other areas of the body. It is capable of delivering dynamic arcs and intensity-modulated radiosurgery.[10] The most recent version is the Novalis TX (Brainlab AG), developed in collaboration with Varian (Palo Alto, CA). It is a dual-energy, dedicated Linac that includes a new micro-Multileaf Collimator (120 leafs, 64 of 2.5-mm width in the center); stereo-Kilovolts imaging; and an onboard imager including cone beam CT-scan. The maximum dose rate is 1000 MU per minute (**Fig. 2**).

A major development brought by the Linac to radiosurgery was the multileaf collimator. It allowed exquisite conformity of the beam to the lesion, taking advantage of the beam's eye-view concept to deliver the beam already with the shape of the tumor. Moreover, the multileaf device allowed introduction of the intensity modulation concept to radiosurgery. Herein, the beam can be modulated by letting the leaf stay more or less time in front of the beam to increase or decrease the intensity of radiation to specific areas of the tumor and areas of normal tissue that need to be spared. More recently, the Linac became capable of intensity-modulation radiation based on time that is taken for delivery of radiation to specific areas, in this way also increasing or decreasing the amount of radiation delivered to determined sites.[31,32] This new approach to intensity modulation is commercially called Rapid Arc (Varian) or VMAT (Elekta, Crowley, UK) depending on the manufacturer of the Linac.

Tomotherapy Hi-Art

The Tomotherapy Hi-Art system (**Fig. 3**) is a Linac combined with a CT-scanner developed in the 1990s as a novel way to deliver dynamic helical radiotherapy. The delivery of the treatment is based on a fan beam and gantry rotation. The treatment is delivered in a helical fashion with continuous and synchronous motion of gantry and couch.[33]

The Tomotherapy Hi-Art is an integrated system for treatment planning, patient set-up, CT-guided treatment, quality assurance, recording, and verification. It was initially proposed for treatment of large-volume tumors and not specifically for radiosurgery. However, it has capabilities for radiosurgery. It has been used to treat with fractionated schemes, delivering low doses to normal tissues because of its high indices of conformity. Tomotherapy is a good option for fractionated stereotactic radiotherapy treatments, decreasing the side effects of conventional radiotherapy. A head ring is used for immobilization, but not for localization. A CT scan is promptly acquired before each treatment and compared with the planning CT scan to ensure precision and correct for tumor evolution during treatment.

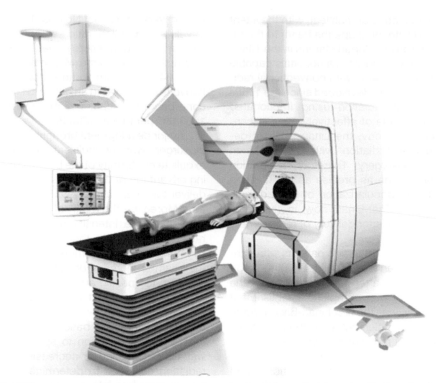

Fig. 2. Novalis TX linear accelerator system features the robotic table, online imaging for localization, including cone-beam CT, oblique X-rays, and infrared system of positioning and monitoring. (*Courtesy of* Brainlab, Feldkirchen, Germany; with permission.)

Cyberknife

The Cyberknife is a 6-MV Linac held by a robot that positions it at different directions to strategically deliver a multitude of beams to cover the complete extent of the lesion with a volume of radiation (**Fig. 4**). This approach is not based on an isocenter but on painting the lesion with strategically directed beams. The Cyberknife was created at Stanford University, initially with the intent to treat cerebral and spinal pathologies; it was, however, quickly applied to treatment of lesions throughout the body using the radiosurgery technique.[34] This capability has revolutionized radiation oncology with the increasing precision of treatment and less number of fractions of radiation. Cyberknife technology was the first approach to follow movement of organs in the human body.[35] It set the stage for several approaches of treating moving targets, such as gated delivery of radiation and four-dimensional radiosurgery planning and delivery. Gated radiation delivery takes advantage of the possibility of predicting the position of the target during organ movement. Delivery of radiation occurs only when the target reaches the know path of the beam. This approach has the drawback of increasing the time of treatment. The four-dimensional radiosurgery technique takes advantage of monitoring with CT the complete pathway of the tumor and irradiating the volume where the tumor travels, thereby irradiating the tumor and also the surrounding tissue. It

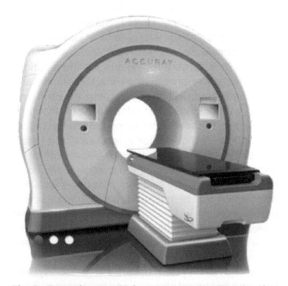

Fig. 3. Tomotherapy High-Art System is a CT-scan platform capable of imaging and delivery treatment in the same setting. (*Courtesy of* Accuray, Sunnyvale, CA; with permission.)

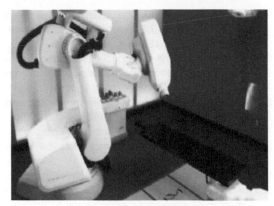

Fig. 4. Cyberknife featuring the robot with six degrees of freedom capable of pointing the linear accelerator to the patient's tumor thereby painting its volume with radiation using multiple nodes (ie, beams). (*Courtesy of* Accuray, Sunnyvale, CA; with permission.)

does, however, accomplish the radiation in a shorter time than gated therapy, paying the price of irradiating more than the tumor volume.

The Cyberknife accomplishes frameless localization with image-acquisition and processing during treatment. A system of oblique digital X-ray images of the patient is compared with previously obtained CT scan images to determine the direction and amount of motion necessary for delivery of radiation precisely to the moving target.[36] In this context, the Cyberknife has been used to treat spine, lung, and abdominal tumors, especially metastases.[35]

SUMMARY

Radiosurgery concepts and techniques transformed neurosurgery and radiation oncology during the end of the twentieth century. The variety of systems gaining space in the market during the last 20 years provides excellent conformity, precision, and versatility to expand this neurosurgery-based technology to multiple specialties in medicine. Now it is used for inoperable tumors in the lung, pancreas, liver, and other sites. Similar to what happened in neurosurgery, the results of stereotactic radiosurgery are appearing in the literature and competing favorably with conventional surgery in a multitude of pathologies. Most likely, other surgeons will also incorporate the radiosurgery technique.

REFERENCES

1. Thime G. Die Bewegungsbestrahlung. Stuttgart (Germany): Verlag; 1959.

2. Leksell L. The stereotaxic method and radiosurgery of the brain. Acta Chir Scand 1951;102:316.

3. Lasak JM, Gorecki JP. The history of stereotactic radiosurgery and radiotherapy. Otolaryngol Clin North Am 2009;42(4):593–9. http://dx.doi.org/10.1016/j.otc. 2009.04.003.

4. Holly FE. Radiosurgery equipment: physical principles, precision, limitations. In: De Salles AA, Goetsch SJ, editors. Stereotactic surgery and radiosurgery. Madison (WI): Medical Physics Publishing Corporation; 1993. p. 185–200.

5. Gorgulho AA, Ishida W, De Salles AA. General imaging modalities: basic principles. In: Lozano AM, Gildenberg PL, Tasker RR, editors. Text book of stereotactic and functional neurosurgery. New York: Springer; 2009.

6. Leksell L. A note on the treatment of acoustic neuromas. Acta Chir Scand 1971;137:763–5.

7. Steiner L, Leksell L, Greitz T, et al. Stereotaxic radiosurgery for cerebral arteriovenous malformations. Report of a case. Acta Chir Scand 1972;138:459–64.

8. De Salles AA, Sedrak M, Lemaire JJ. Future of stereotactic radiosurgery. In: De Salles AA, Gorgulho A, Agazaryan N, et al, editors. Shaped beam radiosurgery: state of the art. 1st edition. Munich: Springer; 2011. p. 307–11.

9. Berkowitz O, Kondziolka D, Bissonette D, et al. The evolution of a clinical registry during 25 years of experience with Gamma Knife radiosurgery in Pittsburgh. Neurosurg Focus 2013;34(1):E4.

10. De Salles AA, Gorgulho A, Selch MT, et al. Radiosurgery from the brain to the spine: 20 years experience. Acta Neurochir Suppl 2008;101:163–8.

11. Hiraoka M, Ishikura SA. Japan clinical oncology group trial for stereotactic body radiation therapy of non-small cell lung cancer. J Thorac Oncol 2007;2(7 Suppl 3):S115–7.

12. Rahman M, Murad GJ, Bova F, et al. Stereotactic radiosurgery and the linear accelerator: accelerating electrons in neurosurgery. Neurosurg Focus 2009;27(3): E13. http://dx.doi.org/10.3171/2009.7.FOCUS09116.

13. Vesper J, Bölke B, Wille C, et al. Current concepts in stereotactic radiosurgery: a neurosurgical and radiooncological point of view. Eur J Med Res 2009; 14:93–101.

14. Levivier M, Gevaert T, Negretti L. Gamma Knife, CyberKnife, TomoTherapy: gadgets or useful tools? Curr Opin Neurol 2011;24(6):616–25. http://dx.doi. org/10.1097/WCO.0b013e32834cd4df.

15. Kjellberg RN, Hanamura T, Davis KR, et al. Brabbpeak proton-beam therapy for arteriovenous malformations. N Engl J Med 1983;309:269–74.

16. Fabrikant JI, Lyman JT, Hosobuchi Y. Stereotactic heavy-ion Bragg peak radiosurgery for intra-cranial vascular disorders: method for treatment of deep arteriovenous malformations. Br J Radiol 1984; 57(678):479–90.

17. Smith A, Gillin M, Bues M, et al. Anderson proton therapy system. Med Phys 2009;36(9):4068–83.

18. Leksell L. Radiosurgery, an operative system. 1978.

19. Kooy HM, Bellerive MR, Loefler JS, et al, editors. Text book of stereotactic and functional neurosurgery. New York: McGraw-Hill Companies; 1998. p. 687–704.

20. Niranjan A, Madhavan R, Gerszten PC, et al. Intracranial radiosurgery: an effective and disruptive innovation in neurosurgery. Stereotact Funct Neurosurg 2012;90:1–7.

21. Thwaites DI, Tuohy JB. Back to the future: the history and development of the clinical linear accelerator. Phys Med Biol 2006;51:R343–62.

22. Friedman WA, Bova FJ. The University of Florida radiosurgery system. Surg Neurol 1989;32(5):334–42.

23. Kjellberg RN, Koehler AM, Preston WM. Intracranial lesions made by bragg peak of a proton beam. In: Haley TJ, Snider RS, editors. Response of the nervous system to ionizing irradiation. Boston: Little, Brown and Company; 1964. p. 36–53.

24. Barcia-Salorio JL, Hernandez G, Broseta J, et al. Radiosurgery treatment of carotid cavernous fistula. Appl Neurophysiol 1982;45:520–2.

25. Betty O, Derechinsky V. Irradiation stéréotaxique multifasceaux. Neurochirurgie 1983;29:295–8.

26. Colombo F, Benedetti A, Pozza F, et al. External stereotactic radiation by linear accelerator. Neurosurgery 1985;16:154–60.

27. Hartmann G, Schlegel W, Sturm V, et al. Cerebral radiation surgery using moving field irradiation at a linear accelerator facility. Int J Radiat Oncol Biol Phys 1985;2:1185–92.

28. Heifetz MD, Wexler M, Thompson R. Single beam radiotherapy knife. A practical theoretical model. J Neurosurg 1984;60:814–8.

29. Winston KR, Lutz W. Linear accelerator as a neurosurgical tool for stereotactic radiosurgery. Neurosurgery 1988;22(3):454–64.

30. Solberg TD, Selch MT, De Salles AA. Fractionated stereotactic radiosurgery: rational and methods. Med Dosim 1998;32(3):209–19.

31. Yu CX. Intensity-modulated arc therapy with dynamic multileaf collimation: an alternative to tomotherapy. Phys Med Biol 1995;40:1435–49.

32. Cardinale RM, Benedict SH, Wu Q, et al. Comparison of three stereotactic radiotherapy techniques: arcs vs. noncoplanar fixed fields vs. intensity modulation. Int J Radiat Oncol Biol Phys 1998;42(2):431–6.

33. Purdie TG, Bissonnette JP, Franks K, et al. Cone-beam computed tomography for on-line image guidance of lung stereotactic radiotherapy: localization, verification, and intrafraction tumor position. Int J Radiat Oncol Biol Phys 2007;68:243–52.

34. Adler J. Frameless radiosurgery. In: De Salles AA, Goetsch SJ, editors. Stereotactic surgery and radiosurgery. Madison (WI): Medical Physics Publishing Corporation; 1993. p. 237–48.

35. Adler JR Jr, Colombo F, Heilbrun MP, et al. Toward an expanded view of radiosurgery [review]. Neurosurgery 2004;55(6):1374–6.

36. Chenery SG, Massoudi F, De Salles AA, et al. Clinical experience with the Cyberknife at Newport radiosurgery center. Radiosurgery 1999;3:34–40.

Stereotactic Radiosurgery of Intracranial Meningiomas

Bruce E. Pollock, MD[a,b,*], Scott L. Stafford, MD[b],
Michael J. Link, MD[a]

KEYWORDS

- Complications • Meningioma • Stereotactic radiosurgery

KEY POINTS

- Meningiomas are typically well visualized on magnetic resonance imaging, facilitating complete radiosurgical coverage.
- A tumor margin dose from 12 to 15 Gy provides a high rate of tumor control and a low complication rate for well-selected patients with World Health Organization (WHO) grade I intracranial meningiomas. Higher doses are typically used when safe for patients with WHO grade II or III meningiomas.
- Tumor control is higher for WHO grade I meningiomas ($\approx 95\%$ at 5 years) compared to WHO grade II ($\approx 60\%$ at 5 years) and 10% for WHO grade III ($\approx 10\%$ at 5 years) meningiomas.
- Increasing tumor volume, prior or concurrent external beam radiation therapy, and location are important predictors of radiation-related complications. Meningiomas of the skull base or tentorium have a lower risk of radiation-related complications compared with convexity or falx meningiomas.

INTRODUCTION

Meningiomas are the most common nonglial tumor affecting the central nervous system. Although meningiomas have been described by earlier neurosurgeons, it was not until Cushing and Eisenhardt in 1938 detailed the clinical presentation, pathology, and surgical treatment that these tumors were more clearly understood.[1] Based on the work and teachings of Dr Cushing, surgical excision became the preferred treatment for patients with symptomatic, intracranial meningiomas. In 1957, Simpson published his landmark article describing 5 grades of meningioma removal that demonstrated the relationship between the aggressiveness of meningioma resection and later tumor recurrences.[2] A grade 1 resection is a complete macroscopic tumor removal with excision of its dural attachments and adjacent abnormal bone. Grade 2 is a complete macroscopic tumor removal with coagulation of its dural attachments. Grade 3 is a complete macroscopic removal of the tumor without resection or coagulation of its dural attachments or extradural extensions. Grades 4 and 5 are partial tumor resection and simple decompression, respectively. The rate of symptomatic meningioma recurrence was 9%, 19%, and 29% for patients having grades 1, 2, and 3 resections, respectively. Simpson concluded that surgery for intracranial meningiomas should be as extensive as possible, understanding that complete tumor removal is often not feasible for many skull-based tumors or for patients with tumors attached to the venous sinuses. Over the past 50 years, neurosurgeons have embraced this attitude, creating the foundation used in the management of meningioma patients.

Advances in anesthesia, neuroimaging, and microsurgical techniques have increased the number of patients having complete resection of

Disclosures: The authors have nothing to disclose.
[a] Department of Neurological Surgery, Mayo Clinic College of Medicine, Rochester, MN, USA; [b] Department of Radiation Oncology, Mayo Clinic College of Medicine, Rochester, MN, USA
* Corresponding author. Department of Neurological Surgery, Mayo Clinic, Rochester, MN 55905.
E-mail address: pollock.bruce@mayo.edu

their meningiomas with acceptable morbidity. However, some meningiomas invade the adjacent neurovascular structures and cannot be completely removed.[3–5] Consequently, most neurosurgeons now recommend subtotal (nonradical) tumor resections for critically located meningiomas as a method to reduce symptomatic mass effect at less risk than a complete tumor resection.[6–10] Nevertheless, even when a meningioma has been completely removed, the tumor recurrence rates may be as high as 15% at 5 years.[11–13] For patients with benign meningiomas (World Health Organization [WHO] grade I) having tumor recurrence or progression, external beam radiation therapy (EBRT) has been used for many years as a postoperative adjunct to provide tumor growth control, and also for patients with atypical (WHO grade II) or malignant (WHO grade III) meningiomas.[9,14–17] Numerous studies have documented that postoperative EBRT decreases tumor recurrence and improves survival for patients after incomplete meningioma resection. Despite improving progression-free survival (PFS) for meningioma patients, EBRT requires 5 to 6 weeks and can result in cognitive decline, radiation-induced neoplasms, or pituitary insufficiency.

As an alternative to surgical resection or EBRT, stereotactic radiosurgery (SRS) has been used for more than 30 years for patients with intracranial meningiomas.[18–22] In this article, the tumor control and complication rates for patients with intracranial meningiomas having single-fraction SRS at the authors' center from 1990 until 2008 are discussed.

INDICATIONS AND TECHNIQUE

The treatment options for patients with intracranial meningiomas include observation with serial imaging, microsurgical resection, EBRT, and SRS. When used appropriately, each modality is important in the management of meningioma patients, and it is not uncommon that a combination of these approaches is needed to achieve tumor control. Factors that are considered in deciding the appropriate treatment include tumor size, tumor location, prior surgery, tumor grade, and patient preference.

Patients with large tumors and symptomatic mass effect are generally considered poor candidates for SRS and surgical resection is performed whenever feasible. Conversely, patients diagnosed with small tumors, especially those patients with minimal deficits, can be considered for observation with serial imaging. Oya and colleagues[23] from the Cleveland Clinic reported 244 patients (277 tumors) who were managed conservatively (mean follow-up, 3.8 years) for their intracranial meningioma. Of note, when volumetric analysis was performed, 114 of 154 tumors (74%) showed tumor enlargement. Factors associated with tumor growth included age ≤60 years, lack of calcification, hyperintensity on T2-weighted magnetic resonance imaging (MRI), tumor size greater than 25 mm, and adjacent edema. Hashimoto and colleagues[24] performed volumetric analysis on 113 patients with incidentally discovered meningiomas. During a mean follow-up period of 46.9 months, 71 tumors (63%) showed a volume increase ≥15%. Tumors located at the skull base grew less frequently (40% vs 75%) and had a longer doubling time when compared with non-skull-base meningiomas (161 months vs 112 months). However, the follow-up period in these studies (approximately 4 years) is too short to conclude that observation alone will be effective for most meningioma patients whose life expectancy when diagnosed is often 20 to 30 years.

If resection is performed and complete tumor removal is not possible, a decision must be made postoperatively either to follow patients with serial MRI or to proceed directly to some form of radiation treatment. Recent studies have shown high rates of tumor progression within 5 to 15 years of subtotal benign meningioma surgery.[10–12] Therefore, it is likely that most patients in their 50s and 60s with WHO grade I meningiomas and definable tumor remnants on postoperative MRI will show tumor growth postoperatively. Patients with a WHO grade II meningioma and residual tumor should be evaluated for either EBRT or SRS. Patients with residual tumor that is more diffuse are typically best suited for EBRT, whereas patients with more nodular tumor remnants can be managed well with SRS. Patients with WHO grade III meningiomas should undergo postoperative EBRT, with SRS being used primarily as a salvage therapy if the patient has progressive tumor enlargement after EBRT.

Radiosurgery at the Mayo Clinic (Rochester, MN) is performed with the Leksell Gamma Knife (Elekta Instruments, Norcross, GA). Dose planning is primarily performed using stereotactic MRI. In recent years, stereotactic CT has been used in addition to MRI for patients with skull-base meningiomas. Modern SRS software facilitates the creation of conformal dose plans that minimize the radiation exposure to adjacent normal structures (**Fig. 1**). Dose prescription must take into account the tumor size, location, histology, and history of prior radiation therapy. Tumor margin doses of 12 to 15 Gy are typically prescribed for patients with presumed or documented WHO grade I

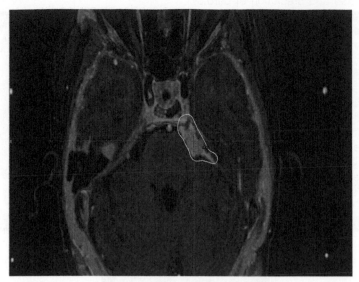

Fig. 1. Radiosurgical dose plan for a left-sided petroclival meningioma. The image is a fusion of a postgadolinium SPGR (Spoiled Gradient Recalled Acquisition in Steady State) MRI and computed tomography. Twelve isocenters of radiation were used to cover a volume of 2.3 cm³. The tumor margin dose was 14 Gy.

meningiomas.[19,21] Higher radiation doses are generally given to patients with WHO grade II or III meningiomas if they have not received prior EBRT and the tumor volume is less than 10 cm³. The radiation dose to the optic apparatus must be considered in patients with tumors in the parasellar region. Doses of 10 to 12 Gy can be given safely to small segments (2–4 mm³) of the optic nerve and chiasm in a single fraction.[25] **Table 1** outlines the type and number of single fraction meningioma SRS cases performed at the Mayo Clinic from 1990 to 2008.

After the procedure, MRI is requested at 6, 12, and 24 months. If there has been no evidence of tumor progression by 24 months, then MRI is generally performed every 2 to 3 years. The tumor size is compared to the imaging performed on the day of SRS. Tumor enlargement greater than 2 mm of the irradiated tumor is considered in-field progression. Tumor growth adjacent to the irradiated tumor is considered marginal progression. Also recorded are radiation-related complications, such as edema (**Fig. 2**), cysts (**Fig. 3**), radiation-induced cavernous malformations (**Fig. 4**),[26,27] and cerebral infarction.

RADIOSURGERY OF WHO GRADE I MENINGIOMAS

Most studies on meningioma SRS have analyzed a heterogenous group of patients that include patients with radiation-induced meningiomas, patients with multiple meningiomas, and patients with neurofibromatosis. Therefore, the understanding of SRS for patients with sporadic, benign intracranial meningiomas is confounded by inclusion of these varied groups into the analysis of tumor control. Moreover, patients who received either prior or concurrent EBRT are also frequently included in the analysis of RRC. To determine the tumor control rate and identify factors associated with RRC after single-session SRS for patients with either presumed intracranial meningiomas or patients with histologically confirmed WHO grade I tumors, the authors' experience for patients treated between 1990 and 2008 at the Mayo Clinic was recently reviewed.[21,28] Four hundred sixteen patients were identified with sporadic, benign intracranial meningiomas with at least 12 months of follow-up after SRS (median, 60 months). Most tumors

Table 1
Meningioma radiosurgery at Mayo Clinic, 1990–2008 (n = 602)[a]

Tumor Type	No. of Patients (%)
Presumed	256 (42.5%)
WHO Grade I	225 (37.4%)
WHO Grade II	39 (6.5%)
WHO Grade III	15 (2.5%)
Radiation-induced	28 (4.7%)
Multiple meningiomas	23 (3.8%)
Neurofibromatosis type II	16 (2.7%)

[a] Meningiomas represented 13.9% of total radiosurgical series (n = 4341).

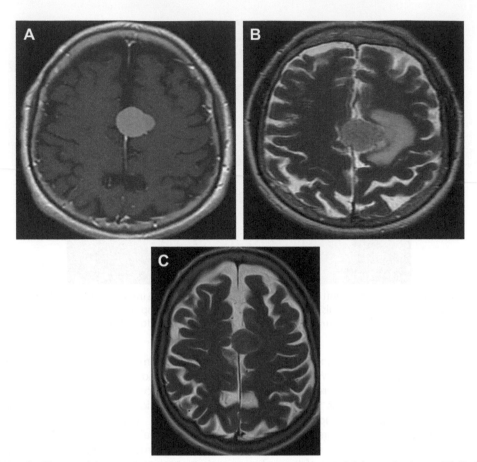

Fig. 2. MRI of a 63-year-old woman with an enlarging, incidentally discovered falx meningioma. (*A*) Gadolinium-enhanced MRI performed before SRS. The treatment volume was 7.2 cm³. The tumor margin dose was 15 Gy. (*B*) T2-weighted MRI performed 7 months after SRS. The patient had a seizure and was started on dexamethasone and anticonvulsant medications. (*C*) T2-weighted MRI performed 4 years after SRS. The tumor has decreased in size and the adjacent edema has resolved. She is seizure-free and has discontinued her anticonvulsant therapy.

(81%) involved the skull base or tentorium. The median tumor volume was 7.3 cm³; the median tumor margin dose was 16 Gy.

Twelve patients (2.9%) died of tumor or treatment-related causes at a median of 60 months (range, 40–122) after SRS. The 5-year and 10-year disease-specific survival (DSS) rate was 97% and 94%, respectively. Multivariate testing found increasing patient age ($P = .01$), prior surgical resection ($P = .005$), and patients with tumors located in the parasagittal/falx/convexity regions ($P = .005$) were negative risk factors for DSS.

Overall, 275 tumors (66.1%) decreased in size and 117 tumors were unchanged (28.1%) for a crude local tumor control (LC) rate of 94%. In-field tumor progression was noted in 11 patients (2.6%) at a median of 43 months after SRS (range, 31–150) (**Fig. 5**). Marginal tumor progression was noted in 13 patients (3.1%) at a median of 74 months after SRS (range, 6–107). The 5-year

and 10-year LC rate was 96% and 89%, respectively. Multivariate analysis found male gender ($P = .03$), prior surgery ($P = .002$), and patients with tumors located in the parasagittal/falx/convexity regions ($P = .02$) to be risk factors for local tumor progression. Of note, 10-year LC rate for patients having SRS for presumed meningiomas was 99.4%.

Forty-five patients (11%) developed permanent RRC at a median of 9 months after SRS (range, 1–125). The 1-year, 5-year, and 10-year RRC rate was 6%, 11%, and 13%, respectively. Multivariate analysis showed increasing tumor volume ($P = .008$) and patients with tumors of the parasagittal/falx/convexity regions ($P = .005$) were associated with permanent RRC. It is worth noting that 3 patients (0.7%) died of RRC after SRS. Two patients died of progressive neurologic deficits and one patient died of status epilepticus. All 3 patients were older (68, 71, and 76 years old,

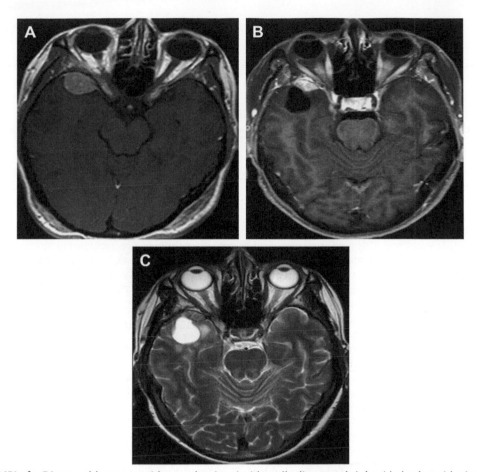

Fig. 3. MRI of a 54-year-old woman with an enlarging, incidentally discovered right-sided sphenoid wing meningioma. (*A*) Gadolinium-enhanced MRI performed at the time of SRS. The treatment volume was 5.8 cm³. The tumor margin dose was 16 Gy. (*B, C*) Gadolinium-enhanced and T2-weighted MRI performed 11 years after SRS. The patient remains asymptomatic and the tumor has decreased in size, but a cyst has developed adjacent to the tumor.

respectively) and had larger tumors (17.0, 25.0, and 30.7 cm³) located in the falx/parasagittal region. No patient developed a radiation-induced tumor after SRS.

Overall, 350 patients (84%) in the series had LC without neurologic morbidity after SRS. The chance of a successful outcome after benign meningioma SRS was greatest for patients with small-volume (<4.0 cm³), unoperated skull-base or tentorial meningiomas (94%). Conversely, patients with large-volume (>12.9 cm³) recurrent tumors of the parasagittal/falx/convexity regions had the lowest chance of LC without neurologic morbidity (25%).

RADIOSURGERY OF WHO GRADE II OR III MENINGIOMAS

In 2000 and 2007, the WHO revised the pathologic grading of meningiomas using a combination of objective criteria (mitotic index) and subjective criteria.[29,30] These changes have resulted in a higher percentage of intracranial meningiomas being classified as WHO grade II (atypical). For example, less than 5% of meningiomas were classified as atypical in the large series (936 tumors) reported by Kallio and colleagues[31] in 1992, whereas Willis and colleagues[32] (314 tumors) noted greater than 20% of meningiomas resected from 1994 until 2003 met the WHO criteria of grade II. The percentage of patients having anaplastic meningiomas (WHO grade III) has remained relatively stable (approximately 1%–2%).

Patients with residual or recurrent WHO grade II or III intracranial meningiomas represent a significant management challenge. Pasquier and colleagues[17] reported 82 patients with WHO grade II meningiomas who received EBRT (mean dose, 54.6 Gy) following initial resection or at the time of recurrence. The 5-year PFS rate for these patients

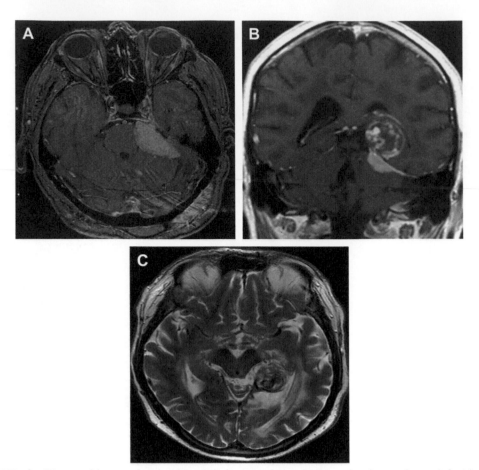

Fig. 4. MRI of a 75-year-old man who developed diplopia and was discovered to have a large, left-sided petro-clival meningioma. (*A*) Gadolinium-enhanced MRI performed at the time of SRS. The treatment volume was 28.9 cm^3. The tumor margin dose was 13 Gy. (*B, C*) Gadolinium-enhanced and T2-weighted MRI performed 7 years after SRS. The tumor is decreased in size, but a new 2-cm mass has developed in the adjacent left temporal lobe causing edema and local mass effect. The patient has not developed any new symptoms related to this lesion.

was 62%. A high mitotic rate was associated with a lower PFS. Rosenberg and colleagues[33] reviewed 13 patients with WHO grade III meningiomas and reported a median survival of 3.4 years despite resection, EBRT, and SRS. Kondziolka and colleagues[20] noted that 83% of WHO grade III meningiomas (24 of 29 tumors) progressed at a median of 15 months after SRS.

Between 1990 and 2008, 54 patients with histologically confirmed WHO grade II (n = 39) or grade III (n = 15) tumors had single-fraction SRS at the authors' center.[34] Four patients were lost to follow-up. In the remaining 50 patients, 27 (54%) were men and most patients (n = 35, 70%) had tumors located in the parasagittal or convexity regions. Four patients (8%) had radiation-induced meningiomas. Importantly, 20 patients (40%) had enlarging tumors (WHO grade II, n = 12; WHO grade III, n = 8) despite having prior EBRT (median dose, 54.0 Gy).

Four patients (WHO grade II, n = 3; WHO grade III, n = 1) had multiple tumors (median, 2 tumors) treated at the time of their initial SRS. The median tumor volume was 14.6 cm^3 (range, 1.8–97.7). The median tumor margin dose was 15.0 Gy (range, 9–20) Four patients with WHO grade II tumors and 3 patients with WHO grade III tumors received concurrent EBRT (median dose, 50.4 Gy). Nine patients underwent repeat SRS at a median of 24 months (range, 7–147) for tumor progression. The median tumor volume was 2.3 cm^3 (range, 1.5–31.0). The median tumor margin dose was 18.0 Gy (range, 14–20). Overall, the 50 patients underwent a total of 61 SRS procedures to treat 71 tumors.

Twenty-two patients (44%) died at a median of 27 months (range, 6–166) after SRS. Nineteen patients (38%) died of tumor progression. The DSS at 1 year and 5 years was 90% and 62%, respectively. Univariate analysis found tumor grade (*P* = .008) to correlate with DSS. The

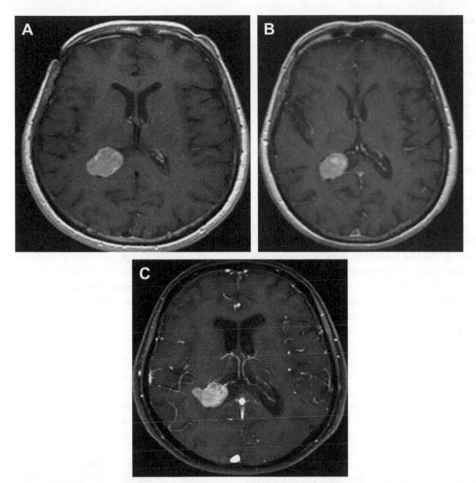

Fig. 5. MRI of a 69-year-old woman with an enlarging right intraventricular meningioma. (*A*) Gadolinium-enhanced MRI performed at the time of SRS. The tumor volume was 7.7 cm^3. The tumor margin dose was 15 Gy. (*B*) Gadolinium-enhanced MRI performed 10 years after SRS shows the tumor to be smaller. (*C*) Gadolinium-enhanced MRI 12.5 years after SRS shows growth on the lateral aspect of the tumor. The patient remained asymptomatic.

1-year and 5-year DSS for patients with a WHO grade II meningioma was 97% and 80%, respectively, compared to 69% and 27% for patients with WHO grade III meningiomas. Multivariate analysis found having failed prior EBRT (*P* = .02) and tumor volume greater than 14.6 cm^3 (*P* = .01) were negative predictors of DSS (see **Fig. 2**). The best DSS was for patients who had not undergone prior EBRT and who had tumor volumes ≤14.6 cm^3. For this subset of 19 patients, DSS was 100% at 1 year and 89% at 5 years. In contrast, the worst DSS was for patients who had failed prior EBRT and had tumor volumes greater than 14.6 cm^3. For these 11 patients, DSS was 55% at 1 year and 15% at 5 years.

Seventy-one tumors (WHO grade II, n = 55; WHO grade III, n = 16) were evaluated by MRI after SRS. Thirty-four (48%) showed local tumor progression. LC was 85% at 1 year and 45% at 5 years. Multivariate analysis found having failed prior EBRT (*P* = .001) and tumor volume greater than 14.6 cm^3 (*P* = .02) were negative predictors of LC. Distant tumor progression was noted in 15 patients (30%). The PFS at 1 year and 5 years was 76% and 40%, respectively. Multivariate analysis found having failed prior EBRT (*P* = .002) was a negative predictor of PFS.

Thirteen patients (26%) developed RRC at a median of 6 months (range, 2–63) after SRS. Of these 13 patients, 7 had undergone either prior EBRT (n = 5) or concurrent EBRT (n = 2). Nine patients (18%) had major complications and 4 patients (8%) had minor complications. The incidence of RRC after SRS was 21% at 1 year and 23% at 5 years. No tested factor correlated with RRC after SRS.

SUMMARY

Single-fraction SRS has been proven to be an important treatment option for patients with intracranial meningiomas. Patient selection is critical for successful meningioma SRS. Factors related to tumor control and RRC include histologic grade, history of prior surgery or EBRT, tumor volume, and tumor location.

REFERENCES

1. Cushing H, Eisenhardt L, editors. Meningiomas: their classification, regional behavior, life history, and surgical end results. Springfield (IL): Charles C. Thomas; 1938.
2. Simpson D. The recurrence of intracranial meningiomas after surgical treatment. J Neurol Neurosurg Psychiatry 1957;20:22–39.
3. Kotapka MJ, Kalia KK, Martinez AJ, et al. Infiltration of the carotid artery by cavernous sinus meningioma. J Neurosurg 1994;81:252–5.
4. Larson JJ, van Loveren HR, Balko G, et al. Evidence of meningioma infiltration into cranial nerves: clinical implications for cavernous sinus meningiomas. J Neurosurg 1995;83:596–9.
5. Sen C, Hague K. Meningiomas involving the cavernous sinus: histological factors affecting the degree of resection. J Neurosurg 1997;87:535–43.
6. Abdel-Aziz KM, Froelich SC, Dagnew E, et al. Large sphenoid wing meningiomas involving the cavernous sinus: conservative surgical strategies for better functional outcomes. Neurosurgery 2004; 54:1375–84.
7. Couldwell WT, Kan P, Liu JK, et al. Decompression of cavernous sinus meningioma for preservation and improvement of cranial nerve function. Technical note. J Neurosurg 2006;105:148–52.
8. Di Maio S, Ramanathan D, Garcia-Lopez R, et al. Evolution and future of skull base surgery: the paradigm of skull base meningiomas. World Neurosurg 2012;78:260–75.
9. Dufour H, Muracciole X, Metellus P, et al. Long-term tumor control and functional outcome in patients with cavernous sinus meningiomas treated by radiotherapy with or without previous surgery: is there an alternative to aggressive tumor removal? Neurosurgery 2001;48:285–96.
10. Klink DF, Sampath P, Miller NR, et al. Long-term visual outcome after nonradical microsurgery in patients with parasellar and cavernous sinus meningiomas. Neurosurgery 2000;47:24–32.
11. Mathiesen T, Lindquist C, Kihlström L, et al. Recurrence of cranial base meningiomas. Neurosurgery 1996;39:2–9.
12. Stafford SL, Perry A, Suman VJ, et al. Primarily resected meningiomas: outcome and prognostic factors in 581 Mayo Clinic patients, 1978 through 1988. Mayo Clin Proc 1998;73:936–42.
13. Sughrue ME, Kane AJ, Shangari G, et al. The relevance of Simpson grade I and II resection in modern neurosurgical treatment of World Health Organization grade I meningiomas. J Neurosurg 2010;113: 1029–35.
14. Goldsmith BJ, Wara WM, Wilson CB, et al. Postoperative irradiation for subtotally resected meningiomas. A retrospective analysis of 140 patients treated from 1967 to 1990. J Neurosurg 1994;80: 195–201.
15. Metellus P, Batra S, Karkar S, et al. Fractionated conformal radiotherapy in the management of cavernous sinus meningiomas: long-term functional outcome and tumor control at a single institution. Int J Radiat Oncol Biol Phys 2010;78:836–43.
16. Slater JD, Loredo LN, Chung A, et al. Fractionated proton radiotherapy for benign cavernous sinus meningiomas. Int J Radiat Oncol Biol Phys 2012; 83:e633–7.
17. Pasquier D, Bijmolt S, Veninga T, et al. Atypical and malignant meningioma: outcome and prognostic factors in 119 irradiated patients. A multicenter, retrospective study of the Rare Cancer Network. Int J Radiat Oncol Biol Phys 2008;71:1388–93.
18. Colombo F, Casentini C, Cavedon C, et al. Cyberknife radiosurgery for benign meningiomas: short-term results in 199 patients. Neurosurgery 2009;64: A7–13.
19. Kollová A, Liscak R, Novotny J, et al. Gamma knife surgery for benign meningioma. J Neurosurg 2007; 107:325–36.
20. Kondziolka D, Mathieu D, Lunsford LD, et al. Radiosurgery as definitive management of intracranial meningiomas. Neurosurgery 2008;62:53–60.
21. Pollock BE, Stafford SL, Link MJ, et al. Single-fraction radiosurgery of benign intracranial meningiomas. Neurosurgery 2012;71:604–13.
22. Santacroce A, Waller M, Régis J, et al. Long-term tumor control of benign intracranial meningiomas after radiosurgery in a series of 4565 patients. Neurosurgery 2012;70:32–9.
23. Oya S, Kim S, Sade B, et al. The natural history of intracranial meningiomas. J Neurosurg 2011;114: 1250–6.
24. Hashimoto N, Rabo CS, Okita Y, et al. Slower growth of skull base meningiomas compared with non-skull base meningiomas based on volumetric and biologic studies. J Neurosurg 2012;116:574–80.
25. Stafford SL, Pollock BE, Leavitt JA, et al. A study on the radiation tolerance of the optic nerves and chiasm after stereotactic radiosurgery. Int J Radiat Oncol Biol Phys 2003;55:1177–81.
26. Kurita H, Sasaki T, Kawamoto S, et al. Chronic encapsulated expanding hematoma in association with gamma knife stereotactic radiosurgery for a

cerebral arteriovenous malformation. Case report. J Neurosurg 1996;84:874–8.

27. Motegi H, Kuroda S, Aoyama H, et al. De novo formation of cavernoma after radiosurgery for adult cerebral arteriovenous malformation. Case report. Neurol Med Chir (Tokyo) 2008;48:397–400.

28. Pollock BE, Stafford SL, Link MJ, et al. Single-fraction radiosurgery for presumed intracranial meningiomas: efficacy and complications from 22-year experience. Int J Radiat Oncol Biol Phys 2012;83:1414–8.

29. Louis DN, Scheithauer BW, Budka H, et al. Meningiomas. In: Kleihues P, Cavenee WK, editors. Pathology and genetics of tumours of the nervous system. Lyon (France): IARC press; 2000. p. 176–84.

30. Perry A, Louis DN, Scheithauer BW, et al. Meningeal Tumors. In: Louis DN, Ohgaki H, Wiestler OD, et al,

editors. WHO classification of tumours of the central nervous system. Lyon (France): IARC press; 2007. p. 164–72.

31. Kallio M, Sankila R, Hakulinen T, et al. Factors affecting operative and excess long-term mortality in 935 patients with intracranial meningioma. Neurosurgery 1992;31:2–12.

32. Willis J, Smith C, Ironside J, et al. The accuracy of meningioma grading: a 10-year retrospective audit. Neuropathol Appl Neurobiol 2005;31:141–9.

33. Rosenberg LA, Prayson RA, Lee J, et al. Long-term experience with world health organization grade III (malignant) meningiomas at a single institution. Int J Radiat Oncol Biol Phys 2009;74:427–32.

34. Pollock BE, Stafford SL, Link MJ, et al. Stereotactic radiosurgery of WHO grade II and III intracranial meningiomas: treatment results based on a 22-year experience. Cancer 2012;118:1048–54.

Stereotactic Radiosurgery of Pituitary Adenomas

Roman Liščák, MD, PhD[a],*, Jana Ježková, MD, PhD[b],
Josef Marek, MD, DrSc[b]

KEYWORDS

- Radiosurgery • Gamma knife • Pituitary adenoma • Hypopituitarism

KEY POINTS

- Radiosurgery is mainly used after transsphenoidal surgery for residual or recurrent tumors.
- The minimum distance required between the secreting adenomas and the optic pathway should be 2 mm; in cases of nonsecreting adenomas this distance is even lower.
- An antiproliferative effect is achieved by radiosurgery in more than 90% of patients.
- The rate of biochemical remission of hypersecreting adenomas is comparable with the results of transsphenoidal surgery, but requires a latency of several years.
- A mean dose of less than 15 Gy applied to the hypophysis can avoid the risk of hypopituitarism after radiosurgery in 97% of patients.

INTRODUCTION

Pituitary adenomas are frequently occurring tumors that, according to the meta-analysis estimate, have a prevalence rate of 16.7%. Furthermore, unexpected expansions in the pituitary (incidentalomas) have been found in 22.5% of patients in magnetic resonance imaging (MRI) and computed tomography studies, with 78% of this number being adenomas.[1] In a series of pituitary incidentalomas that required surgery, pituitary adenomas were diagnosed in 91% of patients.[2] Pituitary adenomas may either be classified according to their size or by their functional status. Pituitary microadenomas are defined as intrasellar adenomas less than 1 cm in diameter; pituitary macroadenomas are those equal to or larger than 1 cm in diameter. Pituitary adenomas may also be categorized as either hypersecretory (functioning) or nonfunctioning.

Treatment of pituitary adenomas is a complex issue, involving neurosurgical, pharmacologic, and radiation treatment modalities. Functioning pituitary adenomas of any size are always referred for treatment because of the risks associated with hypersecretion of hormones. Nonfunctioning pituitary microadenomas should be managed conservatively. Whenever significant changes in tumor size (especially in tumors approaching the chiasm) or alteration of pituitary function are detected, active treatment is recommended. The most common first-line treatment of pituitary tumors is transsphenoidal neurosurgery, which immediately relieves hormonal hypersecretion or the compression of critical structures, leading to the preservation, and in some cases also to the improvement, of visual function, and of impaired pituitary function.[3,4] However, complete tumor removal is not possible in every case, so postoperative fractionated radiotherapy is frequently recommended. Recurrence after postoperative fractionated radiotherapy has been observed in 12.5% to 20% of patients.[5–8]

Disclosures: The authors have nothing to disclose.
[a] Stereotactic and Radiation Neurosurgery, Na Homolce Hospital, Roentgenova 2, Prague 5, 150 30, Czech Republic; [b] Third Department of Internal Medicine, First Faculty of Medicine, Charles University, U Nemocnice 1, 128 08, Prague, Czech Republic
* Corresponding author.
E-mail address: roman.liscak@homolka.cz

Neurosurg Clin N Am 24 (2013) 509–519
http://dx.doi.org/10.1016/j.nec.2013.05.005
1042-3680/13/$ – see front matter © 2013 Elsevier Inc. All rights reserved.

The risk of a secondary brain tumor after fractionated radiotherapy was reported in 1.6% to 2.7% of patients,[5,9,10] and hypopituitarism can develop in 50% to 80% of patients after fractionated radiotherapy for a pituitary adenoma.[11–13] Hormonal normalization is achieved with a latency of 5 to 15 years after conventional fractionated radiation.[14] Given the high incidence of the development of hypopituitarism and the recurrence rate, the indication of adjuvant postoperative radiotherapy has been gradually reassessed.[15] At present, stereotactic radiosurgery (SRS) is preferred to fractionated radiotherapy, provided the anatomic situation allows the indication of this treatment modality.

RADIOSURGERY OF PITUITARY ADENOMAS

The aim of SRS for pituitary adenomas is to stop tumor growth, to normalize the hormonal hypersecretion, and to preserve normal pituitary function and the neurologic function of important structures surrounding the sella turcica, especially the optic nerve.

The historical course of pituitary radiosurgery has covered 6 decades. Charged particle beams were used on the first series of patients treated for pituitary adenomas. However, this technique was available only in special scientific research centers and, for most patients, radiosurgery using heavy charged particles has been limited to 4 world centers (Berkeley, California; Cambridge, Massachusetts; and Moscow and St Petersburg, Russia).[16–18] The domain of linear accelerators is fractionated radiotherapy with limited applications for pituitary SRS.[19,20]

The optimal tool for pituitary SRS nowadays is the gamma knife model C or Perfexion (Elekta Instrument AB, Stockholm) because of the space distribution of the cobalt-60 radiation sources. In previous models (before 1988), the gamma ray sources were distributed in an almost hemispherical array, but the cobalt-60 sources in newer versions of this device are distributed in a toroidal fashion, which makes the dose decrease steeper in a vertical direction (ie, between the chiasma and optic tract and the pituitary adenoma). The relationship of adenoma to the optic tract is the most crucial limit for SRS in this anatomic localization. The steepness of the radiation dose decrease against critical structures can be enhanced by plugging radiation source segments emitting gamma rays that pass through the structures.

A typical plan for SRS achieves the maximal conformity of the marginal dose with the shape of the tumor but also spares the surrounding critical structures such as the optic pathway and any remaining normal pituitary gland tissue. The radiation dose necessary to stop tumor growth (antiproliferative effect) is lower than the dose necessary to achieve normalization of hormonal hypersecretion.[21,22] We typically try to deliver a marginal dose for nonsecreting adenomas (usually on the 50% isodose line) of up to 20 Gy and, for hypersecreting adenomas, of 35 Gy, which makes the indication criteria for SRS stricter for functioning pituitary adenomas. Therefore, SRS is appropriate when a distance of at least 2 mm between a functioning pituitary adenoma and the optic chiasm is guaranteed. This distance is less vital for the SRS of nonfunctioning adenomas. If the target volume of a nonsecreting adenoma is only in contact with the optic pathway over a short section, it is possible to apply a lower isodose to the narrow part of the adenoma that is touching the optic pathway compared with the rest of the adenoma, keeping the dose to the optic pathway under safe limits. Symptomatic compression of the optic pathway is a contraindication for SRS for 2 reasons. First, the shrinkage and the decompression of the optic pathway are not guaranteed in all patients. Second, the loss of vision as a consequence of optic pathway compression is an urgent problem, whereas shrinkage of the adenoma after SRS may require several years. Thus, the final dose selection must take into account the tolerance of the surrounding structures, and the marginal dose is lowered appropriately when necessary.

The optic pathway is the most sensitive structure and the radiation dose should not exceed 8 Gy,[23,24] although in the midterm period (patients with malignant disease and limited life expectancy) a dose of up to 15 Gy can be tolerated.[25] For pituitary radiosurgery planning it is reasonable to consider the optic pathway as more vulnerable where there has been previous conventional fractionated radiotherapy, previous compression, and neurosurgery; this applies to most patients referred for SRS. By contrast, if SRS is the primary treatment, it is possible, while exercising caution, to consider the untouched optic pathway without compression to be more resilient. In such circumstances, a dose of 10 Gy can sometimes be applied to the optic pathway if only a small volume of the critical structure is irradiated. In contrast, in cases with a prior history of radiotherapy, the dose to the optic nerve should be adequately reduced and we do not recommend exceeding 3 Gy in such a situation.

The dose to the brain stem should be kept to less than 14 Gy, the mean dose to the normal pituitary gland to less than 15 Gy, and the dose to the distal infundibulum to less than 17 Gy.[26,27] Compared with the optic pathway, brain stem, pituitary gland, and infundibulum, the other surrounding structures are more radioresistant. Their proximity to the adenoma does not usually limit the SRS. The oculomotor nerves that pass through the cavernous sinus tolerate radiation doses of up to 40 Gy without developing permanent cranial nerve injury.[24]

Concerning pharmacologic treatment shortly before and during SRS, some investigators have reported that the administration of hormone suppression therapy, such as somatostatin analogues or dopaminergic agonists, during irradiation decreased the success of the treatment.[21,28–30] Although the radioprotective effect of somatostatin analogues and dopamine agonists (DAs) was not generally accepted,[31] it was suggested that the administration of DAs should be discontinued for 2 months, the short-acting form of octreotide for 2 weeks, and long-acting somatostatin analogues for 4 months before SRS. Data concerning these withdrawal periods were not experimentally verified in detail. The treatment can be restarted 1 week after SRS.

NONFUNCTIONING PITUITARY ADENOMAS

The main aim of SRS for nonfunctioning pituitary adenomas is to stop tumor growth. According to the published results, an antiproliferative effect of SRS has been achieved in most patients, ranging from 87% to 100%. The median or the mean of the minimum marginal dose has been reported to range from 14 to 16.6 Gy.[26,32–38] Although some centers prefer lower doses to avoid complications, tumor growth after low-dose SRS has been observed. We prefer higher doses, because in our experience the antiproliferative effect is achieved more reliably and we have not observed a higher incidence of complications. For the treatment of nonfunctioning pituitary adenomas, a marginal dose of 20 Gy is usually used. This dose is reduced with large adenomas, after previous fractionated radiotherapy, or in the case of close adenoma contact with the chiasm. The minimum single-session antiproliferative dose on the adenoma margin is described as being 12 Gy; a dose lower than 10 Gy can lead to failure of SRS.[39,40]

In our study we evaluated the results of 79 patients treated for nonfunctioning pituitary adenomas who were followed for at least 3 years (median 5 years).[41] Tumor growth control was achieved in all patients, and in 89% of patients the tumor volume was reduced by an average of 60% of the pretreatment volume. Shrinkage of the adenoma was usually observed 2 years after SRS, although ongoing shrinkage has been seen for years after the procedure (**Fig. 1**). The adenoma was in contact with the chiasm in 15 patients. In all cases the size of the adenoma decreased and it moved away from the chiasm. No visual field defect was found in the irradiated patients and, in 8% of patients, visual improvement was detected.

ACROMEGALY

Treatment of acromegaly is a complex issue, using neurosurgical, pharmacologic, and radiation modalities. Surgery performed by an experienced surgeon can remove 80% to 90% of microadenomas, and 50% of macroadenomas.[42–44] Repeat surgery of pituitary adenomas tends to be less successful compared with the first surgical attempt. For patients with residual and persistent hormonal activity after surgery, treatment options include pharmacologic suppression, irradiation, and a combination of these approaches. The disadvantage of pharmacologic treatment is the necessity for lifelong administration, resulting in high treatment costs. Less financially demanding dopaminergic agonists can only lower insulinlike growth factor I (IGF-I) and growth hormone (GH) levels in a small number of patients: bromocriptine in 10%[45] and cabergoline in one-third of patients.[46] Furthermore, their effect is particularly dependent on initial hormonal activity.[46] Somatostatin analogues are reported to be effective in 22% to 79% of patients.[47–50] The most successful treatment, with GH receptor antagonist pegvisomant, is also the most expensive, and long-term experience of its effect on the growth of pituitary adenomas is lacking.[51,52]

In our study,[53] we followed the results of 96 patients. Of these, 74% had undergone neurosurgery before SRS, and 12.5% had also been irradiated conventionally before SRS. Within 3, 5, and 8 years after SRS, the criterion of being well controlled (GH ≤ 1 μg/L in the oral glucose tolerance test [oGTT] and normal IGF-I according to sex and age) was achieved in 28.6%, 44.2%, and 57.1% respectively. The criterion of being within safe limits (GH <2.5 μg/L with no regard to IGF-I) was achieved in 47.1%, 67.4%, and 85.7% respectively. The criterion of according to IGF-I levels (normal IGF-I levels according to sex and age with no regard to GH) was achieved in 41.1%, 55.8%, and 71.4% of patients respectively. Fifty percent of patients achieved a mean GH of less than 2.5 μg/L within 42 months, normalized their IGF-I within 54 months, and achieved suppression in oGTT GH less than or equal to 1 μg/L with normal IGF-I within 66 months. The effectiveness of SRS depended on initial adenoma hormonal activity (GH and IGF-I serum levels), not on the size of the adenoma. Patients with primary neurosurgery followed by SRS had better outcomes than those

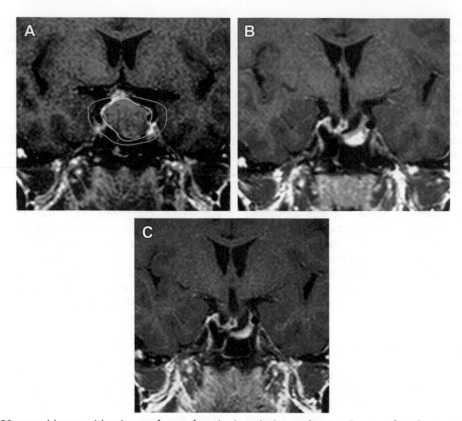

Fig. 1. A 29-year-old man with relapse of a nonfunctioning pituitary adenoma 3 years after the transsphenoidal microsurgery: 50% isodose represents 17 Gy, 23% isodose below the optic chiasm represents 7.8 Gy (*A*); adenoma shrinkage 2 years (*B*) and 5 years after SRS (*C*) (T1-weighted postcontrast sequence).

with SRS only. Irradiation stopped the growth of all adenomas and caused tumor shrinkage in 62.3% of patients (**Fig. 2**).

Any comparison with other published articles is problematic because they vary in their criteria for assessing hormonal normalization, in the length of follow-up, and in the size of groups. Reports in

the literature found GH less than 2.5 μg/L following SRS in 37% to 50% of patients,[54,55] normalization of IGF-I in 15% to 86% of patients,[27,54,56–58] and GH less than or equal to 1 μg/L in the oGTT, and normal IGF-I in 36.9% to 42% of patients.[59,60]

There are only a few reports evaluating the success of conventional fractionated radiotherapy

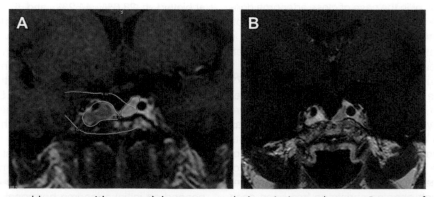

Fig. 2. A 51-year-old women with a growth hormone–producing pituitary adenoma. One year after the neurosurgical operation she underwent SRS, 35 Gy and 8 Gy line imaged, mean dose to the hypophysis (*red*) was 11 Gy (*A*). At checkup 10 years after SRS, the adenoma had regressed, the disease was inactive 2 years after the treatment, and the normal function of hypophysis was preserved (*B*).

with criteria similar to ours. The level of GH less than 2.5 µg/L is reported in 25% to 75% of patients within 5 years and in 21% to 76% of patients within 10 years,[11,12,61,62] and normalization of IGF-I in 2.6% to 60% of patients within 5 years and in 16% to 96% of patients in 10 years and more after conventional radiotherapy.[11,12,61–63] The disadvantage of conventional fractionated radiotherapy is the time required for its therapeutic effect. The effect of the SRS is also slow compared with tumor resection, but is shorter than that of conventional radiotherapy. Until the effect of the irradiation is evident and the hormonal production is normalized, hormonal hypersecretion must be suppressed pharmacologically.

ADRENOCORTICOTROPIC HORMONE–SECRETING PITUITARY ADENOMAS
Cushing Disease

Transsphenoidal surgery is the first line of treatment of Cushing disease, with reported success rates ranging from 64% to 93%.[64,65] Recurrence occurs in 9% to 25% of cases.[65] The treatment options for persistent or recurrent Cushing disease include reoperation, radiotherapy, medical treatment, or bilateral adrenalectomy. After conventional radiotherapy, remission is reported in more than 80% of patients; however, it is associated with a high rate of hypopituitarism along with other complications.[66–68]

Our study group consisted of 26 patients with adrenocorticotropic hormone (ACTH)–secreting pituitary adenomas. The normalization of 24-hour free urinary cortisol was achieved after gamma knife radiosurgery in 46.2%, 65.4%, and 84.6% of patients within 2, 3, and 5 years respectively. The median time to normalization was 2 years. Irradiation stopped the growth of all adenomas and caused tumor shrinkage in 86.7% of patients. In published studies the normalization of 24-hour free urinary cortisol is reported in 28% to 83% of patients after gamma knife radiosurgery.[60,69–71] The time to hormonal normalization was shortest in our patients with Cushing disease compared with acromegaly and prolactinomas. Differences in sensitivity among different types of adenomas have also been observed by other investigators.[72]

Nelson Syndrome

Bilateral adrenalectomy for the treatment of Cushing disease may lead to uncontrolled growth of any preexisting pituitary adenoma because of the negative feedback from endogenous cortisol. Patients with Nelson syndrome have increased ACTH levels; hyperpigmentation; and enlarging, often invasive, pituitary tumors. The treatment options for patients with Nelson syndrome include repeat surgery, conventional fractionated radiotherapy, and SRS. The primary goal of treatment in patients with Nelson syndrome is to prevent further tumor growth. Normalization of hormonal levels is not so crucial, because the target organ (adrenal glands) have been removed so hyperpigmentation is a cosmetic, but not a life-threatening, complication.

Few patients with Cushing disease have to undergo bilateral adrenalectomy in modern times. All our patients were treated by bilateral adrenalectomy before 1989. In our study group, we followed 14 patients with Nelson syndrome. Normal levels of ACTH were only reached in 1 patient. ACTH levels of another 6 patients were approaching the upper levels of the normal limits. After SRS, the adenoma stopped growing or decreased in size in all but 1 patient.

Cessation of growth has been reported in 20 out of 22 cases by Mauermann and colleagues[73] and by Vik-Mo and colleagues[74] in all 10 patients with Nelson syndrome after SRS. Normalization of ACTH is less successful, achieved in only 10% to 36% (14% in our study). However, with the exception of adenoma regrowth, there is at least a decrease in ACTH levels.

Pollock and Young[75] recommended SRS as the initial treatment of most patients with Nelson syndrome, and that this option should be strongly considered for all patients with Cushing disease undergoing bilateral adrenalectomy who have a definable pituitary tumor. In contrast, Vik-Mo and colleagues[74] did not advocate irradiating the sellar region routinely after bilateral adrenalectomy but advised waiting for an increase in the activity of the adenoma at the MRI and ACTH analysis. They argued that only half of patients undergoing bilateral adrenalectomy develop a growing pituitary tumor.

PROLACTINOMA

Pharmacologic treatment with DAs is the treatment of choice for prolactinoma. These drugs normalize prolactin levels and significantly reduce tumor volume in most patients.[76,77] Drug resistance, manifesting as a failure to normalize prolactin levels, was reported in 10% to 20% of microadenomas and 25% to 40% of macroadenomas treated with bromocriptine,[77–79] and in 4% to 10% of microadenomas and 17% to 23% of macroadenomas treated with cabergoline.[80–83] The size of the adenoma was not affected in one-third of bromocriptine-treated patients or in 5% to 10% of cabergoline-treated patients.[84] Drug intolerance was reported in 12% of patients receiving bromocriptine and in only 3% of patients receiving cabergoline.[85,86]

Surgical treatment is indicated for patients who are resistant to pharmacologic therapy or have visual loss. Other indications are pituitary apoplexy causing neurologic symptoms, cystic macroprolactinomas causing clinical symptoms, and intolerance of DA.

SRS is used in patients with resistant prolactinomas, intolerance of DA, and attempts to reduce the dosage or shorten the administration of DA. In macroadenomas in which DA had little or no effect on tumor size reduction, irradiation is given with the aim of decreasing the size of the adenoma.

Our study population consisted of 35 patients with prolactin-secreting pituitary adenomas (9 microadenomas and 26 macroadenomas). SRS resulted in normal serum prolactin levels in 37.1% of these patients who discontinued DA treatment after radiation and in 42.9% of patients who continued DA treatment after radiation. Thus, a total of 80% of patients achieved normal prolactin levels after SRS. Normoprolactinemia after discontinuation of DA was achieved 1 year after SRS in 5.7% of patients, 2 years in 9.1%, 5 years in 20.7%, and 8 years in 50% of patients monitored. The median time to prolactin normalization after discontinuation of DA was 96 months. After achieving normoprolactinemia, no relapse of hyperprolactinemia was observed in any patient. Following SRS, 6 patients became pregnant, which had not been possible before SRS while on DAs because of persistent hyperprolactinemia. After SRS, the prolactinoma stopped growing or decreased in size in all but 1 patient (97.1%). The size of the adenoma decreased even in those patients in whom it had not been changed by previous DA treatment.[87]

Reports in the literature found a normalization of prolactin levels following SRS in 0% to 83% of patients.[19,21,26,29,30,35,55,88,89] The success rate in the treatment of prolactinomas using conventional fractionated radiotherapy has been reported to range from 12.5% to 62.5%.[90–93]

HYPOPITUITARISM AFTER RADIOSURGERY

In the literature, the most common side effect associated with radiation treatment of the sellar region is hypopituitarism. With regard to the development of hypopituitarism after conventional fractionated radiotherapy, the total absorbed dose to the hypothalamo-pituitary axis is the major factor determining the risk and speed of radiation-induced hypopituitarism.[67] It has been observed that the somatotrophic axis is the most radiosensitive, followed by the gonadal,

adrenocortical, and thyroid-stimulating hormone axes. Furthermore, the more the pituitary function is disturbed before conventional radiotherapy, the greater the incidence of hypopituitarism. The incidence of hypopituitarism increases with time after irradiation[67,94] and is reported in 50% to 80% of patients followed up 10 years after conventional irradiation.[11–13] A high number of pituitary deficiencies are reported even in recent studies of fractionated stereotactic radiotherapy. Schalin-Jantti and colleagues[95] referred to the development of new hypopituitarism in 40% of patients during a mean follow-up of 5.2 years; Roug and colleagues[96] reported development of hypopituitarism in 29% of patients with a median of 48 months after this treatment.

Hypopituitarism is a late effect of single-fraction SRS and patients with pituitary adenoma are usually at risk of hypopituitarism 4 or more years after irradiation.[21,27]

The incidence of hypopituitarism following SRS has not been clearly determined. Published data vary widely, ranging from 0% to 40%,[26,32,37,38] but the low incidence of hypopituitarism in a series with short follow-up cannot be considered as a conclusive information. We recorded a high incidence of hypopituitarism in our first patients treated by gamma knife (in 38.2% of patients with acromegaly, 14.3% of patients with prolactinoma, 11.1% of patients with Cushing disease, and 16.7% of patients with Nelson syndrome). This finding led us to analyze the factors that induce the development of hypopituitarism.

In our first published study concerning the development of hypopituitarism, the most important factor was the mean dose to the pituitary gland. If this dose did not exceed 15 Gy, no impairment of thyroid and gonadal function was observed, increasing to 18 Gy for adrenocortical function.[27] A radiation dose of 15 Gy was therefore determined as the maximum safe limit for the mean radiation dose to the pituitary gland. Another factor that influenced the development of hypopituitarism was the maximal dose to the distal infundibulum. Pretreatment factors such as previous neurosurgery, previous partial pituitary deficiency, and tumor volume were shown to play a less important role in the development of hypopituitarism.

The aim of our subsequent study was to verify that hypopituitarism does not develop if the mean dose to the pituitary is less than 15 Gy, and to evaluate the influence of the maximum dose to the distal infundibulum on the development of hypopituitarism.[26] Our study group consisted of 85 patients with pituitary adenomas. The patients were divided in 2 subgroups: the first subgroup consisted of 45 patients who were irradiated with a mean dose to the pituitary of less than 15 Gy. The second subgroup consisted of 40 patients who were irradiated with a mean dose to the pituitary of more than 15 Gy. Hypopituitarism after gamma knife treatment developed in only 1 (2.2%) patient irradiated with a mean dose to pituitary of less than 15 Gy, in contrast with 72.5% of patients irradiated with a mean dose to the pituitary of more than 15 Gy. The radiation dose to the distal infundibulum was an independent factor for the development of hypopituitarism, with a calculated maximum safe dose of 17 Gy. The study published by Feigl and colleagues[32] also showed that the dose to the pituitary stalk was significantly greater in patients with deterioration of pituitary function compared with those in whom this function remained unchanged.

Hypopituitarism as a late effect of radiation can develop many years after irradiation. However, according to our experience, hypopituitarism develops mainly within 4 to 5 years after irradiation. Keeping the mean radiation dose to the pituitary to less than 15 Gy and the dose to the distal infundibulum to less than 17 Gy can significantly decrease the risk of hypopituitarism following SRS.

OTHER SIDE EFFECTS FOLLOWING RADIOSURGERY

In our group of patients, the risk of optic neuropathy was 1%.[41] All patients in whom the deterioration of perimetry (homonymous hemianopia) was detected underwent conventional fractionated irradiation before SRS. Sheehan and colleagues[37] summarized this risk in 35 published series covering the treatment of 1621 patients and reported a similar risk of optic neuropathy (1%) after SRS. The risk of damage to the oculomotor, trochlear, or abducens nerves in the cavernous sinus is less than 1%, and diplopia is frequently a temporary complication.[37,41] Changes detected on MRI in the hypothalamic and temporal regions related to gamma knife treatment were also described in less than 1% of patients. However, most of these patients underwent conventional fractionated radiation before radiosurgery, thus this complication represented a cumulative risk of both treatment methods.[37] Therefore, special caution is required for patients who have undergone conventional fractionated radiotherapy before SRS. As far as vascular injury is concerned, carotid artery stenosis was reported in only 2 cases.[21] To date, radiation-induced neoplasm has not been published after SRS of pituitary adenoma.

SUMMARY

Radiosurgery is an integral part of the treatment approach to pituitary adenomas.[97] It is mainly used after transsphenoidal surgery for residual or recurrent tumors. The radiation dose necessary to stop tumor growth (antiproliferative effect) is lower than the dose that is necessary to achieve normalization of hormonal hypersecretion. An antiproliferative effect is achieved by radiosurgery in more than 90% of patients. The rate of biochemical remission of hypersecreting adenomas is comparable with the results of transsphenoidal surgery, but requires a latency of several years. A mean dose of less than 15 Gy applied to the hypophysis and a dose to the distal part of infundibulum of less than 17 Gy can avoid the risk of hypopituitarism after radiosurgery in 97% of patients.

REFERENCES

1. Ezzat S, Asa S, Couldwell W, et al. The prevalence of pituitary adenomas. Cancer 2004;101:613–9.
2. Freda PU, Post KD. Differential diagnosis of sellar masses. Endocrinol Metab Clin North Am 1999; 28:81–117, vi.
3. Nomikos P, Ladar C, Fahlbusch R, et al. Impact of primary surgery on pituitary function in patients with non-functioning pituitary adenomas-a study on 721 patients. Acta Neurochir (Wien) 2004;146: 27–35.
4. Oyesiku NM, Tindall GT. Endocrine-inactive adenomas: surgical results and prognosis. In: Landolt AM, Vance ML, Reilly PL, editors. Pituitary adenomas. New York: Churchill Livingstone; 1996. p. 377–83.
5. Breen P, Flickinger JC, Kondziolka D, et al. Radiotherapy for nonfunctional pituitary adenoma: analysis of long-term tumor control. J Neurosurg 1998;89:933–8.
6. Ebersold MJ, Quast LM, Laws ER Jr, et al. Long term results in transsphenoidal removal of nonfunctioning pituitary adenomas. J Neurosurg 1986;64:713–9.
7. Flickinger JC, Nelson PB, Martinez AJ, et al. Radiotherapy of non-functional adenomas of the pituitary gland. Cancer 1989;63:2409–14.
8. Salmi J, Grahne B, Valtonen S, et al. Recurrence of chromophobe pituitary adenomas after operation and postoperative radiotherapy. Acta Neurol Scand 1982;66:681–9.
9. Brada M, Ford D, Ashley S, et al. Risk of second brain tumor after conservative surgery and radiotherapy for pituitary adenoma. BMJ 1992; 304(6838):1343–6.
10. Tsang RW, Brierley JD, Panzarella T, et al. Radiation therapy for pituitary adenoma: treatment outcome

and prognostic factors. Int J Radiat Oncol Biol Phys 1994;30:557–65.

11. Barrande G, Pittino-Lungo M, Coste J, et al. Hormonal and metabolic effects of radiotherapy in acromegaly: long-term effect of 128 patients followed in a single center. J Clin Endocrinol Metab 2000;85:3779–85.

12. Biermasz NR, van Dulken H, Roelfsema F. Postoperative radiotherapy in acromegaly is effective in reducing GH concentration to safe levels. Clin Endocrinol 2000;53:321–7.

13. Minniti G, Jaffrain-Rea M, Osti M, et al. The long-term efficacy of conventional radiotherapy in patients with GH-secreting pituitary adenomas. Clin Endocrinol 2005;62:210–6.

14. Landolt AM, Haller D, Lomax A, et al. Stereotactic radiosurgery for recurrent surgically treated acromegaly: comparison with fractionated radiotherapy. J Neurosurg 1998;88:1002–8.

15. Lillehei KO, Kirschman DL, Kleinschmidt-DeMasters BK, et al. Reassessment of the role of radiation therapy in the treatment of endocrine-inactive pituitary macroadenomas. Neurosurgery 1998;43:432–9.

16. Kjellberg RN, Abe M. Stereotactic Bragg peak proton beam therapy. In: Lunsford LD, editor. Modern stereotactic neurosurgery. Boston: Martinus Nijhoff Publishing; 1988. p. 463–71.

17. Levy RP, Fabrikant JI, Frankel KA. Heavy charged particle radiosurgery of the pituitary gland: clinical result of 840 patients. Stereotact Funct Neurosurg 1991;57:22–35.

18. Linfoot JA, Lawrence JH, Born JL, et al. The alpha particle or proton beam in radiosurgery of the pituitary gland for Cushing's disease. N Engl J Med 1963;269:597–601.

19. Mitsumori M, Shrieve DC, Alexander E 3rd, et al. Initial clinical results of LINAC-based stereotactic radiosurgery and stereotactic radiotherapy for pituitary adenomas. Int J Radiat Oncol Biol Phys 1998; 42:573–80.

20. Voges J, Sturm V, Deuss U, et al. LINAC-radiosurgery in pituitary adenomas: preliminary results. Acta Neurochir Suppl 1996;65:41–3.

21. Pollock BE, Nippoldt TB, Stafford SL, et al. Results of stereotactic radiosurgery in patients with hormone-producing pituitary adenomas: factors associated with endocrine normalization. J Neurosurg 2002; 97:525–30.

22. Vladyka V, Liščák R, Šimonová G, et al. Gamma knife radiosurgery of pituitary adenomas. Results in the group of 163 patients treated during the last five years. Čas Lék Česk 2000;139:757–66 [in Czech].

23. Leber KA, Bergloff J, Pendl G. Dose response tolerance of the visual pathways and cranial nerves of the cavernous sinus to stereotactic radiosurgery. J Neurosurg 1998;88:43–50.

24. Tishler RB, Loeffler JS, Lunsford LD, et al. Tolerance of cranial nerves of the cavernous sinus to radiosurgery. Int J Radiat Oncol Biol Phys 1993;27: 215–21.

25. Liščák R, Vladyka V. Radiosurgical hypophysectomy in painful bone metastasis from breast cancer. Čas Lék Česk 1998;137:154–7 [in Czech].

26. Marek J, Ježková J, Hána V, et al. Is it possible to avoid hypopituitarism after irradiation of pituitary adenomas by the Leksell gamma knife? Eur J Endocrinol 2011;164:169–78.

27. Vladyka V, Liščák R, Novotný J Jr, et al. Radiation tolerance of functioning pituitary tissue in gamma knife surgery for pituitary adenomas. Neurosurgery 2003;52:309–17.

28. Landolt AM, Haller D, Lomax N, et al. Octreotide may act as a radioprotective agent in acromegaly. J Clin Endocrinol Metab 2000;85:1287–9.

29. Landolt AM, Lomax N. Gamma knife radiosurgery for prolactinomas. J Neurosurg 2000;93(Suppl 3): 14–8.

30. Pouratian N, Sheehan J, Jagannathan J, et al. Gamma knife radiosurgery for medically and surgically refractory prolactinomas. Neurosurgery 2006; 59:255–64.

31. Castinetti F, Taieb D, Kuhn JM, et al. Outcome of gamma knife radiosurgery in 82 patients with acromegaly: correlation with initial hypersecretion. J Clin Endocrinol Metab 2005;90:4438–88.

32. Feigl GC, Bonelli CM, Berghold A, et al. Effects of gamma knife radiosurgery of pituitary adenomas on pituitary function. J Neurosurg 2002;97(Suppl 5): 415–21.

33. Iwai Y, Yamanaka K, Yoshioka K. Radiosurgery for non-functioning pituitary adenomas. Neurosurgery 2005;56:699–705.

34. Losa M, Valle M, Mortini P, et al. Gamma knife surgery for treatment of residual non-functioning pituitary adenomas after surgical debulking. J Neurosurg 2004;100:438–44.

35. Petrovich Z, Yu C, Gianotta SL, et al. Gamma knife radiosurgery for pituitary adenoma: early results. Neurosurgery 2003;53:51–61.

36. Pollock BE, Carpenter PC. Stereotactic radiosurgery as an alternative to fractionated radiotherapy for patients with recurrent or residual non-functioning pituitary adenomas. Neurosurgery 2003;53:1086–94.

37. Sheehan JP, Niranjan A, Sheehan JM, et al. Stereotactic radiosurgery for pituitary adenomas: an intermediate review of its safety, efficacy, and role in the neurosurgical treatment armamentarium. J Neurosurg 2005;102(4):678–91.

38. Wowra B, Stummer W. Efficacy of gamma knife radiosurgery for non-functioning pituitary adenomas: a quantitative follow up with magnetic resonance imaging-based volumetric analysis. J Neurosurg 2002;97(Suppl 5):429–32.

39. Ganz JC. Gamma knife treatment of pituitary adenomas. Stereotact Funct Neurosurg 1995; 64(Suppl 1):3–10.

40. Thorén M, Rähn T, Guo WY, et al. Stereotactic radiosurgery with the cobalt-60 gamma-unit in the treatment of growth hormone-producing pituitary tumors. Neurosurgery 1991;29:663–8.

41. Liščák R, Vladyka V, Marek J, et al. Gamma knife radiosurgery for endocrine-inactive pituitary adenomas. Acta Neurochir 2007;149: 999–1006.

42. Freda PU, Wardlaw SL, Post KD. Long-term endocrinological follow-up evaluation in 115 patients who underwent transsphenoidal surgery for acromegaly. J Neurosurg 1998;89:353–8.

43. Kreutzer J, Vance ML, Lopes MB, et al. Surgical management of GH-secreting pituitary adenomas: an outcome study using modern remission criteria. J Clin Endocrinol Metab 2001;86:4072–7.

44. Swearingen B, Barker FG 2nd, Katznelson L, et al. Long-term mortality after transsphenoidal surgery and adjunctive therapy for acromegaly. J Clin Endocrinol Metab 1998;83:3419–26.

45. Jaffe CA, Barcan AL. Treatment of acromegaly with dopamine agonists. J Clin Endocrinol Metab 1992; 21:713–35.

46. Abs R, Verhelst J, Maiter D, et al. Cabergoline in the treatment of acromegaly: a study in 64 patients. J Clin Endocrinol Metab 1998;83:374–8.

47. Baldelli R, Colao A, Razzore P, et al. Two-year follow-up of acromegalic patients treated with slow release lanreotide (30 mg). J Clin Endocrinol Metab 2000;85:4099–103.

48. Bevan JS, Atkin SL, Atkinson AB, et al. Primary medical therapy for acromegaly: an open, prospective, multicenter study of the effects of subcutaneous and intramuscular slow-release octreotide on growth hormone, insulin-like growth factor I, and tumor size. J Clin Endocrinol Metab 2002; 87:4554–63.

49. Newman CB, Melmed S, Snyder PJ, et al. Safety and efficacy of long term octreotide therapy of acromegaly: results of a multicenter trial in 103 patients – a clinical research center study. J Clin Endocrinol Metab 1995;80:2768–75.

50. Vance ML, Harris AG. Long-term treatment of 189 acromegalic patients with somatostatin analog octreotide. Arch Intern Med 1991;151: 1573–8.

51. Trainer PJ, Drake WM, Katznelson L, et al. Treatment of acromegaly with the growth hormone-receptor antagonist pegvisomant. N Engl J Med 2000;342:1171–7.

52. van der Lely AJ, Hutson RK, Trainer PJ, et al. Long-term treatment of acromegaly with pegvisomant, a growth hormone receptor antagonist. Lancet 2001; 358:1754–5.

53. Ježková J, Marek J, Hána V, et al. Gamma knife radiosurgery for acromegaly – long-term experience. Clin Endocrinol 2006;64:588–95.

54. Attanasio R, Epaminonda P, Motii E, et al. Gamma-knife radiosurgery in acromegaly: a 4-year follow-up study. J Clin Endocrinol Metab 2003;88:3105–12.

55. Choi JY, Chang JH, Chang JW, et al. Radiological and hormonal responses of functioning pituitary adenomas after gamma knife radiosurgery. Yonsei Med J 2003;44:602–7.

56. Ikeda H, Jokura H, Yoshimoto T. Transsphenoidal surgery and adjuvant gamma knife treatment for growth hormone-secreting pituitary adenoma. J Neurosurg 2001;95:285–91.

57. Jagannathan J, Sheehan J, Pouratian N, et al. Gamma knife radiosurgery for acromegaly: outcomes after failed transsphenoidal surgery. Neurosurgery 2008;62:1262–70.

58. Vik-Mo EO, Øksnes M, Pedersen PH, et al. Gamma knife stereotactic radiosurgery for acromegaly. Eur J Endocrinol 2007;157:255–63.

59. Castinetti F, Nagai M, Morange I, et al. Long-term results of stereotactic radiosurgery in secretory pituitary adenomas. J Clin Endocrinol Metab 2009; 94:3400–7.

60. Wann H, Chihiro O, Yuan S. MASEP gamma radiosurgery for secretory pituitary adenomas: experience in 347 consecutive cases. J Exp Clin Cancer Res 2009;11:28–36.

61. Cozzi R, Barausse M, Asnaghi D, et al. Failure of radiotherapy in acromegaly. Eur J Endocrinol 2001;145:717–26.

62. Thalassinos NC, Tsagarakis S, Ioannides G, et al. Megavoltage pituitary irradiation lowers but seldom leads to safe GH levels in acromegaly: a long-term follow-up study. Eur J Endocrinol 1998;138:160–3.

63. Barkan AL, Halasz I, Dornfeld KJ, et al. Pituitary irradiation is ineffective in normalizing plasma insulin-like growth factor I in patients with acromegaly. J Clin Endocrinol Metab 1997;82:3187–91.

64. Hammer D, Tyrrell JB, Lamborn KR, et al. Transsphenoidal microsurgery for Cushing's disease: initial outcome and long-term results. J Clin Endocrinol Metab 2004;89:6348–57.

65. Laws ER, Reitmeyer M, Thapar K, et al. Cushing's disease resulting from pituitary corticotrophic microadenoma. Treatment results from transsphenoidal microsurgery and gamma knife radiosurgery. Neurochirurgie 2002;48:294–9.

66. Estrada J, Boronat M, Mielgo M, et al. The long-term outcome of pituitary irradiation after unsuccessful transsphenoidal surgery in Cushing's disease. N Engl J Med 1997;336:172–7.

67. Littley MD, Shalet SM, Beardwell CG. Hypopituitarism following external beam radiotherapy for pituitary tumours in adults. Q J Med 1989;70:145–60.

68. Tsang RW, Brierley JD, Panzarella T, et al. Role of radiation therapy in clinical hormonally-active pituitary adenomas. Radiother Oncol 1996;41:45–53.

69. Höybye C, Grenbäck E, Rähn T, et al. Adrenocorticotropic hormone-producing pituitary tumors: 12- to 22-year follow-up after treatment with stereotactic radiosurgery. Neurosurgery 2001;49(2):284–91.

70. Jagannathan J, Sheehan JP, Pouratian N, et al. Gamma knife surgery for Cushing's disease. J Neurosurg 2007;106:980–7.

71. Sheehan JM, Vance ML, Sheehan JP, et al. Radiosurgery for Cushing's disease after failed transsphenoidal surgery. J Neurosurg 2000;93:738–42.

72. Pollock BE, Brown PD, Nippoldt TB, et al. Pituitary tumor type affects the chance of biochemical remission after radiosurgery of hormone-secreting pituitary adenomas. Neurosurgery 2008;62(6):1271–6.

73. Mauermann WJ, Sheehan JP, Chernavvsky DR, et al. Gamma knife surgery for adrenocorticotropic hormone-producing pituitary adenomas after bilateral adrenalectomy. J Neurosurg 2007;106:988–93.

74. Vik-Mo EO, Øksnes M, Pedersen PH, et al. Gamma knife stereotactic radiosurgery of Nelson syndrome. Eur J Endocrinol 2009;160:143–8.

75. Pollock BE, Young WF Jr. Stereotactic radiosurgery for patients with ACTH-producing pituitary adenomas after prior adrenalectomy. Int J Radiat Oncol Biol Phys 2002;54(3):839–41.

76. Bevan JS, Webster J, Burke CW. Dopamine agonists and pituitary tumor shrinkage. Endocr Rev 1992;13:220–40.

77. Molitch ME, Elton RL, Blackwell RE, et al. Bromocriptine as primary therapy for prolactin-secreting macroadenomas: results of a prospective multicenter study. J Clin Endocrinol Metab 1985;60:698–705.

78. Berezin M, Shimon I, Hadani M. Prolactinoma in 53 men: clinical characteristics and modes of treatment (male prolactinoma). J Endocrinol Invest 1995;18:436–41.

79. Liuzzi A, Dallabonzana D, Oppizzi G, et al. Low doses of dopamine agonists in the long-term treatment of macroprolactinomas. N Engl J Med 1985;313:656–9.

80. Colao A, Di Sarno A, Sarnacchiaro F, et al. Prolactinomas resistant to standard dopamine agonists respond to chronic cabergoline treatment. J Clin Endocrinol Metab 1997;82:876–83.

81. Di Sarno A, Landi ML, Cappabianca P, et al. Resistance to cabergoline as compared with bromocriptine in hyperprolactinemia: prevalence, clinical definition, and therapeutic strategy. J Clin Endocrinol Metab 2001;86:5256–61.

82. Muratori M, Arosio M, Gambino G, et al. Use of cabergoline in the long-treatment of hyperprolactinemic and acromegalic patients. J Endocrinol Invest 1997;20:537–46.

83. Verhelst J, Abs R, Maiter D, et al. Cabergoline in the treatment of hyperprolactinemia: a study in 455 patients. J Clin Endocrinol Metab 1999;84:2518–22.

84. Molitch ME. Dopamine resistance of prolactinomas. Pituitary 2003;6:19–27.

85. Rains CP, Bryson HM, Fitton A. Cabergoline. A review of its pharmacological properties and therapeutic potential in the treatment of hyperprolactinemia and inhibition lactation. Drugs 1995;49:255–79.

86. Webster J. A comparative review of the tolerability profiles of dopamine agonists in the treatment of hyperprolactinemia and inhibition lactation. Drug Saf 1996;14:228–38.

87. Ježková J, Hána V, Kršek M, et al. Use of the Leksell gamma knife in the treatment of prolactinoma patients. Clin Endocrinol 2009;70:732–41.

88. Kim SH, Huh R, Chang JW, et al. Gamma knife radiosurgery for functioning pituitary adenomas. Stereotact Funct Neurosurg 1999;72:101–10.

89. Mokry M, Ramschak-Schwarzer S, Simbrunner J, et al. A six year experience with the postoperative radiosurgical management of pituitary adenomas. Stereotact Funct Neurosurg 1999;72(Suppl 1):88–100.

90. Gómez F, Reyes FI, Faimen C. Nonpuerperal galactorrhea and hyperprolactinemia. Clinical findings, endocrine features and therapeutic responses in 56 cases. Am J Med 1977;62:648–60.

91. Johnston DG, Hall K, Kendall-Taylor P, et al. The long-term effects of megavoltage radiotherapy as sole or combined therapy for large prolactinomas: studies with high definition computerized tomography. Clin Endocrinol 1986;24:675–85.

92. Mehta AE, Reyes FI, Faiman C. Primary radiotherapy of prolactinomas. 8- to 15-year follow-up. Am J Med 1987;83:49–58.

93. Zierhut D, Flentje M, Adolph J, et al. External radiotherapy of pituitary adenomas. Int J Radiat Oncol Biol Phys 1995;33:307–14.

94. Brada M, Rajan B, Traish D, et al. The long-term efficacy of conservative surgery and radiotherapy in the control of pituitary adenomas. Clin Endocrinol 1993;38:571–8.

95. Schalin-Jantti C, Valanne L, Tenhunen M, et al. Outcome of fractionated stereotactic radiotherapy in patients with pituitary adenomas resistant to conventional treatment: a 5.25-year follow up study. Clin Endocrinol (Oxf) 2010;73:72–7.

96. Roug S, Rasmussen AK, Juhler M, et al. Fraction-ated stereotactic radiotherapy in patients with acromegaly: an interim single-centre audit. Eur J Endocrinol 2010;162:685–94.

97. Lunsford LD, Niranjan A, Kobayashi T, et al. Stereo-tactic radiosurgery for patients with pituitary ade-nomas. Practice guideline report #3-04. 2004. Available at: www.IRSA.org/Pituitary Guideline.pdf.

Radiosurgery for Vestibular Schwannomas

Jean Régis, MD[a],*, Romain Carron, MD[b],
Christine Delsanti, MD[b], Denis Porcheron, PhD[a,c],
Jean-Marc Thomassin, MD[d], Xavier Murracciole, MD[c],
Pierre-Hugues Roche, MD[e]

KEYWORDS

- Radiosurgery • Acoustic neuromas • Gamma Knife • Hearing • Facial palsy • Tinnitus • Imbalance

KEY POINTS

- The superior safety of radiosurgery over microsurgery in small to middle-sized vestibular schwannomas (VS) has been demonstrated in 5 prospective comparative studies, all of which used Gamma Knife radiosurgery. Normal facial movement and functional hearing are more likely to be preserved with radiosurgery than with microsurgery.
- For large Koos Stage IV VS, a combined approached with a deliberate subtotal tumor removal and functional monitoring followed by radiosurgery of the remnant reduces the risk of facial nerve palsy in comparison with radical tumor removal.
- Multisession radiosurgery (stereotactic radiotherapy) has not yet been proved to have any advantages over single-session, high-precision radiosurgery.

INTRODUCTION

Within the last 3 last decades, microsurgery and stereotactic radiosurgery (SRS) have become well established management options for vestibular schwannomas (VS). Advancement in the management of VS can be separated into 3 periods: the microsurgical pioneer period; the demonstration of SRS as a first-line therapy for small to medium-sized VS; and, at present, a period of SRS maturity based on a large worldwide patient accrual.

Owing to the young age and the benign nature of the lesion, long life expectancy, and the potential severity of functional risks, in the modern era VS should be managed by experienced multidisciplinary teams who are able to integrate all microsurgical and radiosurgical approaches to provide the highest level of care, the highest probability of functional preservation, and a good quality of life. Modern literature provides us with sufficient evidence that the series must include high patient volumes with sufficiently long-term follow-up. This

Disclosures: The first and corresponding author has to disclose congress sponsoring from Accuray, Brainlab, Elekta, Varian.
[a] Department of Stereotaxic and Functional Neurosurgery, Gammaknife Unit, La Timone University Hospital, Inserm U751, 264, Rue Saint-Pierre 13385 Marseille Cedex 5, France; [b] Department of Stereotaxic and Functional Neurosurgery, Gammaknife Unit, La Timone University Hospital, 264, Rue Saint-Pierre 13385 Marseille Cedex 5, France; [c] Department of Radiation Oncology, La Timone University Hospital, 264, Rue Saint-Pierre 13385 Marseille Cedex 5, France; [d] Department of ENT, Head and Neck Surgery, La Timone University Hospital, 264, Rue Saint-Pierre 13385 Marseille Cedex 5, France; [e] Department of Neurosurgery, Northern University Hospital, 264, Rue Saint-Pierre 13385 Marseille Cedex 5, France
* Corresponding author.
E-mail address: jregis@mail.ap-hm.fr

neurosurgery.theclinics.com

research has enabled us to identify the potential roles and limitations of each technique.

VESTIBULAR SCHWANNOMA RADIOSURGERY

Between July 1992 and June 2011, 3050 VS were operated on in the Department of Functional Neurosurgery of Timone University Hospital in Marseille, France. All 3050 of these patients have been included in the series reported here. Patients were preoperatively evaluated and prospectively followed up with a clinical evaluation including Pure Tone Audiometry (PTA), Speech Discrimination Score (SDS), vestibulometry, Schirmer test, and serial magnetic resonance imaging scans (recommended at 6 months, then at 1, 2, 3, 5, 7, 10, and 15 years). One hundred forty-eight patients had neurofibromatosis type II (NF II). Follow-up of 3 years or more was available for 2336 patients (patients with NF II excluded). The mean age was 66.3 years. Tumor classification according to Koos stage was I (17.6%), II (51.8%), III (27%), and IV (3.6%). Initial symptoms were hypoacusia in 49.5% of patients, tinnitus in 19.4%, and vertigo in 13.2%, while 5.1% experienced instability. A history of sudden hearing loss was reported in 21.5%. Of note, microsurgical resection of the VS had been performed before SRS in 7% of patients. The day before intervention, hypoacusia was reported in 87% of patients, tinnitus in 65%, imbalance in 52%, vertigo in 31%, facial palsy in 8.2%, hemifacial spasm in 7.5%, trigeminal neuralgia in 5.3%, and facial hypoesthesia in 4.8%. The methodology has been previously described.[1]

Defining the limits of the tumor is first done on the stereotactic 3-dimensional T1-weighted gadolinium-enhanced MR sequence. The absence of distortion between the MR and stereotactic computed tomography (CT) scan is systematically checked, and a shift in the dose plan is performed consequently if and when necessary. The limits of the internal auditory canal, vestibule, semicircular canals, and cochlea are defined on CT. Dosimetry corresponding to the cisternal portion of the tumor, and adjacent cochlear and facial nerve, respectively, are corrected according to high-resolution T2-weighted imaging (CISS; Siemens) with and without contrast. The dose to the margin is 12 Gy for patients with poor hearing (Gardner-Robertson ≥3) and 11 Gy if hearing is still serviceable.[2] The dose-selection policy has not changed since 1992 for VS, which confers a very good homogeneity to this series. Patients were treated using a Gamma Knife (GK), models B, 4, 4C, and Perfexion, over this time interval.

CLINICAL OUTCOMES

The prospective cohort of Timone Hospital demonstrates, in the last of neuroimaging (MR) follow-ups, tumor control in 97.5% of the patients. In the patients with continuous growth of the VS at the 3-year mark (2.5%), the authors have consequently been led to propose repeat SRS (20 patients) or a resection (39 patients). MRI follow-up during the first year revealed an average 20% increase in tumor volume, followed thereafter by stabilization at 3 years after radiosurgery. After the third year a decrease in tumor volume was typically observed (**Fig. 1**). At 7 years the volume corresponds to 60% of the volume at time of SRS (40% decrease). The rate of transient facial palsy was less than 0.5%. This rate was 3% during the first period, corresponding to the learning curve (with the first 100 patients). The rate was subsequently reduced to 1.4% during the period

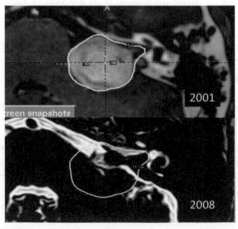
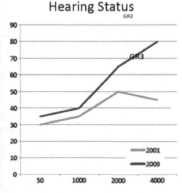

Fig. 1. Example of result of radiosurgery.

preceding the introduction of the workstations (involving 212 patients), and dropped further to 0.5% after the introduction of the dose-planning workstations, and their integration in anatomic imaging (360 patients). Since the introduction of robotization (2319 patients), this rate of transient facial palsy has virtually disappeared in unilateral VS.

In addition, between 2005 and 2010 an extensive search and cross-referencing exercise was conducted on PubMed, which uncovered 213 articles. Of these, 55 reported on a series of more than 30 patients, providing the authors with safety efficacy data. A second filtering enabled the ruling out of any duplicated series and general review articles (15 articles). The majority are retrospective studies. However, 3 studies were prospective, reporting on 69, 78, and 111 patients, respectively.[3–5] The main series reported and their results are summarized in **Table 1**. These series are very heterogeneous in terms of radiation-delivery techniques, size of tumors, doses used, inclusion or exclusion of NF II patients, the number of patients who had been operated on previously, methods of measurement, definition of tumor control, and overall duration of follow-up time, from when the patient is released postsurgery to the final outpatient visit.

The results of the 15 series of GK radiosurgery are fairly homogeneous.[3–16] Only 1 series that used a linear accelerator (LINAC) has been found, in which hearing was not evaluated.[17] In the GK series, tumor control between 3 and 10 years of follow-up ranges from 92% to 98% (97.5% for the present series), with a rate of 90% indicated in the 1 LINAC-based series. Trigeminal injury rates range from 0% to 9% (0.5% in the present series and 3.6% with LINAC). The rate of facial palsy varies between 0% and 7% (0.5% in the present series and 4.4% with LINAC). The rate of serviceable hearing preservation ranges from 56.6% to 78.6% (63% in the present series and no report found with LINAC). No radiation-induced tumor has been reported.

Seven series of stereotactic radiotherapy (SRT) were reviewed and are shown in **Table 2**.[18–24] These reports are fairly heterogeneous in terms of technique. Maire and colleagues[21] report having treated much bigger lesions than the others. The Chang series[19] is hypofractionated (3 fractions, 18–21 Gy). The others are hyperfractionated from 25 to 32 fractions, delivering 45 to 57.6 Gy, by fractions of 1.8 to 2 Gy. In the Andrews series[24] the follow-up is too short to draw any substantial or valid conclusions. In the remaining series, tumor control ranges between 93% and 98%. The rate of injury of the trigeminal nerve varies between 0% and 4.7%. The rate of facial nerve impairment ranges from 0% to 13%. In some reports,[18,20,22] there is no systematic objective evaluation based on preoperative and postoperative PTA and SDS. For example, in the series of Combs and colleagues[20] PTA was performed in only 25% of the patients, and in only 33% for Koh and colleagues.[22] In the series of Chan and colleagues[18] the evaluation of serviceable hearing preservation was based on results from telephone interviews conducted on the patients. Maire and colleagues[21] provide no information regarding hearing outcome. Only 2 articles give an objective assessment on functional hearing, where it was preserved in 56% and 74.3% of the patients, respectively.[19,23] Chan's results showed an average loss in conversational frequencies of 15 dB, compared with 10 dB in the present series of GK radiosurgery.[18] To date, there is no convincing evidence that the rate of functional hearing preservation is superior using SRT in comparison with single-fraction SRS. However, carcinogenesis was reported in 2 of the SRT series, with an incidence of 1.7% and 2.2%.[21,22]

OTHER CONCERNS REGARDING VESTIBULAR SCHWANNOMA RADIOSURGERY
Comparison with Microsurgical Resection

If there is ever a condition whereby the safety and efficacy of SRS compares favorably with microsurgical resection, it is definitely with small to medium-sized VS (Koos I–III). All 5 of the existing comparative studies have reported similar results demonstrating a much lower rate of facial motor nerve impairment, and a much higher rate of serviceable hearing preservation with GK radiosurgery, compared with microsurgical resection.[25–29]

LINAC-Based Vestibular Schwannoma Radiosurgery

To date, the data on LINAC-based VS remains limited, but the series of Friedman and colleagues[17] reports results similar to those for GK radiosurgery, at least in terms of trigeminal and facial nerve complications. A series that would allow a proper evaluation on the quality of hearing outcome following LINAC-based radiosurgery has not yet been performed. Several centers using LINACs have stated their failure in obtaining satisfactory safety results after single-fraction SRS, prompting them to manage patients with VS using either multisession SRS or SRT in the hope of improving their results.

Table 1
Radiosurgery for vestibular schwannomas: analysis of the literature between 2005 and 2010 (Medline), and comparison with present series

Authors,[Ref.] Year	Population/ Previous Surgery	Volume (cm³)	Marginal Dose (Gy)	Follow-Up (mo) Lost to Follow-Up	Tumor Control (%)	V (%)	VII (%)	VIII (%)
Gamma Knife								
Chung et al,[6] 2005 R	195 39%	4.1 (0.04–23.1)	13 (11–18.2)	31 (1–110) 2 lost	At 10 y: 96.8	1.1	1.5	60
Lunsford et al,[8] 2005 R	829 20%	2.5	13 (10–20)	NR >10 y 252 pts	At 10 y: 98	3.1	<1	78.6
Wowra et al,[4] 2005 R	111 33.3%	1.6 (0.08–8.7)	13 (10–16)	7 y (5–9.6)	At 6 y: 95	2.7	2.7	NR
Van Eck et al,[3] 2005 P	78 NR	2.28 (0.1–11.7)	13–20	22	97.4	3.8	1.2	69.2
Hasegawa et al,[7] 2005 R	317 22.7%	5.6 (0.2–36.7) GR 1–2: 30.6%	13.2 (10–18)	93 29 lost	94.4 (10 y: 92)	2	2ᵃ	67.5
Hempel et al,[50] 2006 R	123 NR	1.6 (0.1–9.9)	13 (10–14.5)	98 (63–129)	NR	5.8	0	NR
Liu et al,[10] 2006 R	74 25.6%	10.8 (0.11–27.8)	12.3 (12–14)	68.3 (30–122)	95.9 at 5 & 10 y	7	5	72.3
Hudgins et al,[9] 2006 R	159 NR	3.3	14 (8–20)	12 y	96.4	0	0	NR

Chopra et al,[11] 2007 R	216 / 0%	1.3 (0.08–37.5)	13 (12–13)	68 (max: 143)	98.3 at 10 y	3.7	0	56.6
Niranjan et al,[12] 2008 R	96 / NR	0.112 mm³ (0.1–0.5) Koos I	13 (10–18)	28 (12–144)	99	0	0	63.3
Régis et al,[1,13] 2008 P	184 / 0%	NR GR 1 & 2	12	7 y (3–13)	NR	0.6	0.7	At 3 y: 60
Timmer et al,[5] 2009 P	69 / NR	2.28 (0.02–10.2)	11 (9.3–12.5)	14 (3–56) 16 lost	NR	9	7	75
Kano et al,[15] 2009 R	77 / 0%	0.75 (0.07–7.7) GR 1: 46/GR 2: 31	12.5 (12–13)	20 mo (6–40)	97.4	NR	0	At 1 y 89.3, at 2 y 66.8
Tamura et al,[16] 2009 P	74 / 0%	1.35 (0.06–4.6) GR 1	12 (9–13)	55.6 (3–11 y)	93	NR	0	78.4 at 3 y
Franzin et al,[14] 2009 R	50 / 0%	0.73 (0.03–6.6) GR 1 or 2	13 (12–16)	36 (6–96)	96	NR	0	68
Present series P	2087 / 7%	2.63 GR 1 & 2: 46%	12.3	Minimum 3 y	97.5	0.5	0.5	63
LINAC								
Friedman et al,[17] 2006 R	390 / 20%	NR	12.5 (10–22.5)	40 42 lost	At 5 y: 90	3.6	4.4	NR

Abbreviations: GR, grade; NR, not reported; P, prospective; R, retrospective.

[a] No sufficient follow-up for a serious evaluation.

Data from Refs.[1,3–12,14–17,50]

Table 2
Stereotactic radiotherapy: analysis of the literature between 2005 and 2010 (Medline)

Authors,Ref. Year	Population	Tumor Volume (cm³)	Technique	Follow-Up (mo) Lost to Follow-Up	Tumor Control (%)	V (%)	VII (%)	VIII (%)	Carcinogenesis (%)
LINAC									
Combs et al,[20] 2005 R	106 16%	3.9 (2.7–30.7)	57.6 Gy in 32 fractions 1.8 Gy 6 wk	48.5 (3–172)	At 3 y 94.3 At 5 y 93	4.7	2.3	NR Audiometry 25 Preservation 94	0
Chan et al,[18] 2005a R	70 21%	2.4 (0.05–21.1)	54 Gy in 30 fractions 1.8 Gy 6 wk	45	At 3 y 100 At 5 y 98	4	13	NR	0
Chang et al,[19] 2005 R	61 13%	Diameter mean: 18.5 mm (5–32)	Cyber knife 18–21 Gy in 3 fractions 6–7 Gy, 3 d	48 (36–62)	98.4	0	3.3	74.3 14 dB loss	0
Koh et al,[22] 2007 R	60 NR	4.9 (0.3–49)	X-Knife 50 Gy, 25 fractions 5 wk	31.9 (6.1–107.4)	At 5 y 96.2 (95% CI 91.1–100)	1.6	1.6	NR Audiometry 33 Preservation 77.3	1.7
Andrews et al,[24] 2009 R	89	1.6	48.5 fractions of 1.8 Gy (50.4/46.8)	14.7	97.8b	0b	2.2b	73.3b	0b
Thomas et al,[23] 2007 P	34	1.1 (0.3–9.6)	45 Gy in 25 fractions of 2	36.5 (12–85)	95.7	0	6	56	0
Maire et al,[21] 2006 R	45	NR	50.4 Gy in fractions of 1.8	80 (4–227)	95 (2 dead)	0	0	NR	2.2

Abbreviations: CI, confidence interval; NR, not reported; P, prospective; R, retrospective.

a No audiometry before and after (telephone evaluation only).

b No sufficient follow-up for a proper evaluation.

Data from Refs.[18–24]

Stereotactic Radiotherapy for Vestibular Schwannomas

The rare series of SRT with a solid methodology (more than 3 years of follow-up, minimum number of patients, preoperative and postoperative PTA and SDS) show the rates of trigeminal and facial nerve injuries, as well as functional hearing preservation, as being roughly comparable with those of GK radiosurgery.[18–24] The authors have found no series relying on objective, audiometric data that shows a clear improvement in functional hearing preservation after SRT when compared with GK radiosurgery. Severe, acute sudden hearing losses following SRT have also been reported.[30]

Observation of Vestibular Schwannomas

Simple follow-up (observation) based on clinical interviews and serial MRI scans has been advocated for a significant period. For several years, this has been the standard used by the authors for small intracanalicular VS. Under conditions of sufficiently long periods between follow-ups, combined with strict criteria for defining growth, the vast majority of the modern observational series demonstrate that most tumors will grow and that the majority of patients will, over the course of a few years, progressively lose functional hearing (if hearing was still functional at the commencement of the "wait and see" strategy). Sughrue and colleagues,[31] in a comprehensive review of the literature, reported a total population of 982 patients with follow-up over a period of 26 to 52 months. In this series there was a mean growth of 2.9 mm per year, and 50% of the patients lost functional hearing, despite the short duration of the maximum follow-up relative to life expectancy. In this article the speed of growth is a much more reliable predictor of probability of losing functional hearing than the initial size of the VS. Bakkouri and colleagues[32] published a series detailing 325 patients, and emphasized the difficulties faced in maintaining rigorous patient follow-ups. In fact, Bakkouri reports a tracking loss of 24% of the 325 patients. This loss occurred despite the effort to retain and maintain contact and follow-ups. The authors have recently performed a comparison on this wait-and-see attitude with an early proactive radiosurgical management strategy.[33] This trial has demonstrated ($P = .0009$) that at 3 years, patients who were operated on by GK have a 73.3% chance of preserving functional hearing as opposed to a mere 35% with the simple wait-and-see strategy. Consequently, for these patients radiosurgery is an opportunity to preserve their residual functional hearing. It is to their benefit that radiosurgery is the initial proposal. In another study, the authors focused on patients who had several years with serial audiometry before radiosurgery.[34] Among these 72 consecutive patients, an annual hearing loss of 3.72 dB per year was observed before radiosurgery, 4.06 dB per year the first year after GK surgery and 1.24 dB per year in the following years. This study supports the findings of the authors' previous study, and suggests an early nonsignificant risk of hearing loss corresponding to SRS toxicity, but thereafter a protective effect from SRS. The authors have also successfully demonstrated that in younger patients, the probability of preserving functional hearing is high.[16] These findings have subsequently been confirmed by Lobato and colleagues,[35] which provides additional support in favor of earlier proactive radiosurgical management of these patients.

Management of Large Vestibular Schwannomas

Large Stage IV Koos VS, with significant mass effect on the brainstem, require microsurgical decompression. However, the radical removal of these very large tumors, even in the best hands, can be associated with a major risk of facial palsy (50%–60%). In the authors' experience, only 55% of patients had long-term preservation of normal facial nerve function (House-Brackman 1 or 2) after the radical removal of large Koos Stage IV VS. Consequently, 7 years ago the authors turned away from this approach and moved to a combined approach as standard management for patients with larger Koos Stage IV tumors. The first step of this combined approach is the deliberate, partial removal of the tumor under neuromonitoring of the motor facial nerve. The retrosigmoid approach is used in most cases. The second step is carried out 3 to 6 months following the microsurgery procedure, with radiosurgery being used to treat the residual tumor. This paradigm shift from radical removal to the combined approach has increased the preservation rate of the motor facial function from 55% to 85%. Functional hearing, however, is rarely retained.

With Koos Stage IV, tumors of a reasonable size, generally in patients with a small posterior fossa, and a modest mass effect on the brainstem, can benefit from cautious radiosurgery, especially when the patient's hearing is still functional.[36] The phenomenon of transient increase in VS volume after radiosurgery may cause a decline in the patient's neurologic condition, thus making a resection mandatory.[37,38] However, in the authors' experience, among 95 VS patients with moderate Koos Stage IV tumor at the time of radiosurgery, none has presented such a complication in many years of follow-up. The tumor control rate has been 95% and the functional hearing preservation rate 65%. No patient has developed a facial palsy after SRS.

Young Patient Age

Younger patients have better clinical results after VS SRS, especially in terms of hearing preservation.[16,35] Preserving function, and particularly motor facial function, is of utmost importance in young patients with a long life expectancy, making radiosurgery the preferred surgical method for this population group.

Risk of Secondary Malignancy After Radiosurgery

The risk of secondary malignancy must be factored and discussed whenever younger patients are being treated with ionizing radiation therapy. Recent literature directly pertaining to this issue provides high-quality articles using evidence-based methodology.[39,40] To date, there is no demonstration of an increased risk of carcinogenesis in patients who have undergone single-fraction SRS, meaning that if this risk actually exists then it must be very low, and should be weighed against the risk of perioperative mortality of microsurgery, which statistics place at 1% to 2%. These articles clearly demonstrate that this putative risk must not be regarded as an argument through which a patient may lose out on the benefits gained, and a dramatic reduction of risk, from radiosurgery in comparison with microsurgery. Rowe and colleagues[39] compiled a comparison of the risks of persons having received radiosurgery at some time in their life with those with no history of radiosurgical treatment, through the use of the UK Registry of Causes of Death. In this comparison, no increased risk of cancer was seen in patients who had undergone SRS. According to Cahan and colleagues,[41] the criteria for carcinogenesis can only be discussed if the secondary tumor differs in type from the treated tumor.

Malignant Transformation of Vestibular Schwannomas

The malignant transformation of benign schwannomas, which is extremely rare, is a phenomenon different from carcinogenesis proper (radiation-induced tumors). Within the literature studies, 7 cases of VS, regarded as "benign" at the time of the first surgery, were found to be malignant at the point of second surgery. A key fact is that all of these patients had been exposed to the physical aggression of a surgical resection, but, with regard to radiosurgical interventions, only 5 patients had radiosurgical exposure.[42–44] Comey and colleagues[45] put forth the hypothesis "that the tumors initially regarded as benign, may already contain a minority of malignant components, which subsequently progressed, and led to tumor recurrence and malignant behavior".

Hydrocephalus After Vestibular Schwannoma Radiosurgery

Communicating hydrocephalus can be observed in VS patients. This condition is more frequent in older patients and when the tumor is large. Roche and colleagues[46,47] have demonstrated that there is no increased risk of developing any radiologic or clinical signs of hydrocephalus after SRS.

Management of Vestibular Schwannomas that Fail Radiosurgery

In cases of failure after SRS, if the lesion size is still compatible with SRS, a second radiosurgical procedure is proposed. In the authors' experience, this has a high probability of efficacy.[48] However, in these cases the risk of functional hearing loss is higher compared with patients having initial SRS. When the tumor is too big for a second radiosurgery procedure, the authors always propose a combined approach of nonradical removal followed by a second radiosurgery, and no longer propose the radical removal of VS, owing to the significantly higher rate of facial palsy.[49]

SUMMARY

The authors' series of 2336 patients who underwent GK radiosurgery and were subsequently followed and monitored for more than 3 years demonstrates a high rate of tumor control with a very low risk of trigeminal nerve injury (0.5%) or facial palsy (0.5%). Serviceable hearing preservation stands at 65% after 3 years, but is highly dependent on several factors, including the initial quality of hearing, history of hearing loss, patient's age, and radiation dose to the cochlea at the time of SRS. In favorable cases, the hearing preservation rate can be as high as 90%. When compared with the natural historical course of these tumors, these results are in favor of a protective effect of radiosurgery on hearing. Throughout more than 20 years of experience, no clinical benefit has been demonstrated with either multisession SRS or SRT on comparison with high-precision, single-fraction SRS single-dose radiosurgery for VS.

REFERENCES

1. Régis J, Tamura M, Wikler D, et al. Radiosurgery: operative technique, pitfalls and tips. Prog Neurol Surg 2008;21:54–64.
2. Gardner G, Robertson JH. Hearing preservation in unilateral acoustic neuroma surgery. Ann Otol Rhinol Laryngol 1988;97:55–66.
3. van Eck AT, Horstmann GA. Increased preservation of functional hearing after gamma knife surgery for vestibular schwannoma. J Neurosurg 2005; 102(Suppl):204–6.
4. Wowra B, Muacevic A, Jess-Hempen A, et al. Outpatient gamma knife surgery for vestibular schwannoma: definition of the therapeutic profile based on a 10-year experience. J Neurosurg 2005;102(Suppl):114–8.
5. Timmer FC, Hanssens PE, van Haren AE, et al. Gamma knife radiosurgery for vestibular schwannomas: results of hearing preservation in relation to the cochlear radiation dose. Laryngoscope 2009;119(6):1076–81.
6. Chung WY, Liu KD, Shiau CY, et al. Gamma knife surgery for vestibular schwannoma: 10-year experience of 195 cases. J Neurosurg 2005;102(Suppl): 87–96.
7. Hasegawa T, Fujitani S, Katsumata S, et al. Stereotactic radiosurgery for vestibular schwannomas: analysis of 317 patients followed more than 5 years. Neurosurgery 2005;57(2):257–65 [discussion: 257–65].
8. Lunsford LD, Niranjan A, Flickinger JC, et al. Radiosurgery of vestibular schwannomas: summary of experience in 829 cases. J Neurosurg 2005; 102(Suppl):195–9.
9. Hudgins WR, Antes KJ, Herbert MA, et al. Control of growth of vestibular schwannomas with low-dose Gamma Knife surgery. J Neurosurg 2006; 105(Suppl):154–60.
10. Liu D, Xu D, Zhang Z, et al. Long-term outcomes after Gamma Knife surgery for vestibular schwannomas: a 10-year experience. J Neurosurg 2006; 105(Suppl):149–53.
11. Chopra R, Kondziolka D, Niranjan A, et al. Long-term follow-up of acoustic schwannoma radiosurgery with marginal tumor doses of 12 to 13 Gy. Int J Radiat Oncol Biol Phys 2007;68(3):845–51.
12. Niranjan A, Mathieu D, Flickinger JC, et al. Hearing preservation after intracanalicular vestibular schwannoma radiosurgery. Neurosurgery 2008; 63(6):1054–62 [discussion: 1062–3].
13. Régis J, Tamura M, Delsanti C, et al. Hearing preservation in patients with unilateral vestibular schwannoma after gamma knife surgery. Prog Neurol Surg 2008;21:142–51.
14. Franzin A, Spatola G, Serra C, et al. Evaluation of hearing function after Gamma Knife surgery of vestibular schwannomas. Neurosurg Focus 2009; 27(6):E3.
15. Kano H, Kondziolka D, Khan A, et al. Predictors of hearing preservation after stereotactic radiosurgery for acoustic neuroma. J Neurosurg 2009; 111(4):863–73.
16. Tamura M, Carron R, Yomo S, et al. Hearing preservation after gamma knife radiosurgery for vestibular schwannomas presenting with high-level hearing. Neurosurgery 2009;64(2):289–96 [discussion: 296].
17. Friedman WA, Bradshaw P, Myers A, et al. Linear accelerator radiosurgery for vestibular schwannomas. J Neurosurg 2006;105(5):657–61.
18. Chan AW, Black P, Ojemann RG, et al. Stereotactic radiotherapy for vestibular schwannomas: favorable outcome with minimal toxicity. Neurosurgery 2005;57(1):60–70 [discussion: 60–70].
19. Chang SD, Gibbs IC, Sakamoto GT, et al. Staged stereotactic irradiation for acoustic neuroma. Neurosurgery 2005;56(6):1254–61 [discussion: 1261–3].
20. Combs SE, Volk S, Schulz-Ertner D, et al. Management of acoustic neuromas with fractionated stereotactic radiotherapy (FSRT): long-term results in 106 patients treated in a single institution. Int J Radiat Oncol Biol Phys 2005;63(1):75–81.
21. Maire JP, Huchet A, Milbeo Y, et al. Twenty years' experience in the treatment of acoustic neuromas with fractionated radiotherapy: a review of 45 cases. Int J Radiat Oncol Biol Phys 2006;66(1):170–8.
22. Koh ES, Millar BA, Ménard C, et al. Fractionated stereotactic radiotherapy for acoustic neuroma: single-institution experience at The Princess Margaret Hospital. Cancer 2007;109:1203–10.
23. Thomas C, Di Maio S, Ma R, et al. Hearing preservation following fractionated stereotactic radiotherapy for vestibular schwannomas: prognostic implications of cochlear dose. J Neurosurg 2007; 107(5):917–26.
24. Andrews DW, Werner-Wasik M, Den RB, et al. Toward dose optimization for fractionated stereotactic radiotherapy for acoustic neuromas: comparison of two dose cohorts. Int J Radiat Oncol Biol Phys 2009;74(2):419–26.
25. Pollock BE, Lunsford LD, Kondziolka D, et al. Outcome analysis of acoustic neuroma management: a comparison of microsurgery and stereotactic radiosurgery. Neurosurgery 1995;36(1):215–24 [discussion: 224–9]. [published erratum appears in Neurosurgery 1995;36(2):427].
26. Régis J, Pellet W, Delsanti C, et al. Functional outcome after gamma knife surgery or microsurgery for vestibular schwannomas. J Neurosurg 2002;97(5):1091–100.
27. Myrseth E, Møller P, Pedersen PH, et al. Vestibular schwannomas: clinical results and quality of life

after microsurgery or gamma knife radiosurgery. Neurosurgery 2005;56(5):927–35 [discussion: 927–35].

28. Pollock BE, Driscoll CL, Foote RL, et al. Patient outcomes after vestibular schwannoma management: a prospective comparison of microsurgical resection and stereotactic radiosurgery. Neurosurgery 2006;59(1):77–85 [discussion: 77–85].

29. Myrseth E, Møller P, Pedersen PH, et al. Vestibular schwannoma: surgery or gamma knife radiosurgery? A prospective, nonrandomized study. Neurosurgery 2009;64(4):654–61 [discussion: 661–3].

30. Chang SD, Poen J, Hancock SL, et al. Acute hearing loss following fractionated stereotactic radiosurgery for acoustic neuroma. Report of two cases. J Neurosurg 1998;89:321–5.

31. Sughrue ME, Yang I, Aranda D, et al. The natural history of untreated sporadic vestibular schwannomas: a comprehensive review of hearing outcomes. J Neurosurg 2010;112(1):163–7.

32. Bakkouri WE, Kania RE, Guichard JP, et al. Conservative management of 386 cases of unilateral vestibular schwannoma: tumor growth and consequences for treatment. J Neurosurg 2009;110(4): 662–9.

33. Régis J, Carron R, Park MC, et al. Wait-and-see strategy compared with proactive Gamma Knife surgery in patients with intracanalicular vestibular schwannomas. J Neurosurg 2010;113(Suppl): 105–11.

34. Yomo S, Carron R, Thomassin JM, et al. Longitudinal analysis of hearing before and after radiosurgery for vestibular schwannoma. J Neurosurg 2012;117(5):877–85.

35. Lobato-Polo J, Kondziolka D, Zorro O, et al. Gamma knife radiosurgery in younger patients with vestibular schwannomas. Neurosurgery 2009;65(2):294–300 [discussion: 300–1].

36. Roche PH, Robitail S, Pellet W, et al. Results and indications of gamma knife radiosurgery for large vestibular schwannomas. Neurochirurgie 2004; 50(2-3 Pt 2):377–82 [in French].

37. Nagano O, Serizawa T, Higuchi Y, et al. Tumor shrinkage of vestibular schwannomas after Gamma Knife surgery: results after more than 5 years of follow-up. J Neurosurg 2010;113(Suppl):122–7.

38. Delsanti C, Roche PH, Thomassin JM, et al. Morphological changes of vestibular schwannomas after radiosurgical treatment: pitfalls and diagnosis of failure. Prog Neurol Surg 2008;21:93–7.

39. Rowe J, Grainger A, Walton L, et al. Risk of malignancy after gamma knife stereotactic radiosurgery. Neurosurgery 2007;60(1):60–5 [discussion: 65–6].

40. Ganz JC. Gamma knife radiosurgery and its possible relationship to malignancy: a review. J Neurosurg 2002;97(Suppl 5):644–52.

41. Cahan WG, Woodard HQ, Higinbotham NL, et al. Sarcoma arising in irradiated bone: report of eleven cases. Cancer 1948;1:3–29.

42. Akamatsu Y, Murakami K, Watanabe M, et al. Malignant peripheral nerve sheath tumor arising from benign vestibular schwannoma treated by gamma knife radiosurgery after two previous surgeries: a case report with surgical and pathological observations. World Neurosurg 2010;73(6):751–4.

43. Murakami K, Jokura H, Kawagishi J, et al. Development of intratumoral cyst or extratumoral arachnoid cyst in intracranial schwannomas following gamma knife radiosurgery. Acta Neurochir (Wien) 2011; 153(6):1201–9.

44. Regis J, Muracciole X. Associated is not induced! World Neurosurg 2010;73(6):642–3.

45. Comey CH, McLaughlin MR, Jho HD, et al. Death from a malignant cerebellopontine angle triton tumor despite stereotactic radiosurgery. Case report [see comments]. J Neurosurg 1998;89(4):653–8.

46. Roche PH, Ribeiro T, Soumare O, et al. Hydrocephalus and vestibular schwannomas treated by Gamma Knife radiosurgery. Neurochirurgie 2004; 50(2–3 Pt 2):345–9 [in French].

47. Roche PH, Khalil M, Soumare O, et al. Hydrocephalus and vestibular schwannomas: considerations about the impact of gamma knife radiosurgery. Prog Neurol Surg 2008;21:200–6.

48. Yomo S, Arkha Y, Delsanti C, et al. Repeat gamma knife surgery for regrowth of vestibular schwannomas. Neurosurgery 2008;64:48–54.

49. Fuentes S, Arkha Y, Pech-Gourg G, et al. Management of large vestibular schwannomas by combined surgical resection and gamma knife radiosurgery. Prog Neurol Surg 2008;21:79–82.

50. Hempel JM, Hempel E, Wowra B, et al. Functional outcome after gamma knife treatment in vestibular schwannoma. Eur Arch Otorhinolaryngol 2006;263: 714–8.

Stereotactic Radiosurgery for Nonvestibular Schwannomas

Toshinori Hasegawa, MD

KEYWORDS

- Facial schwannoma • Functional outcomes • Gamma knife • Jugular foramen schwannoma
- Nonvestibular schwannoma • Stereotactic radiosurgery • Trigeminal schwannoma

KEY POINTS

- Stereotactic radiosurgery is one of the reasonable treatment options for patients with small to medium-sized nonvestibular schwannomas without a severe compression of the brainstem.
- Because of tumor origin and surrounding critical structures, it is extremely difficult to completely remove nonvestibular schwannomas without any complications.
- Stereotactic radiosurgery provides a good tumor control for nonvestibular schwannomas.
- Morbidity after stereotactic radiosurgery is much less than that after microsurgery for patients with nonvestibular schwannomas, particularly with facial or jugular foramen schwannomas.

INTRODUCTION

Intracranial schwannomas are generally benign tumors that arise from Schwann cells of the nerve sheath. Most of them originate from eighth cranial nerve, so-called vestibular schwannoma. Nonvestibular schwannomas are rare, accounting for less than 10% of intracranial schwannomas,[1] and less than 0.5% of all intracranial neoplasms.[2] Complete tumor resection is the desirable curable approach for these benign tumors. However, it is not always feasible to achieve complete resection without any complications, even for experienced neurosurgeon using recent microsurgical techniques as well as neuromonitoring, because of the tumor origin and surrounding critical structures such as cranial nerves, vessels, and brainstem. Also, the rarity of nonvestibular schwannomas would be one of the reasons why complete resection without worsening of neurologic function is extremely difficult. Accordingly, a relatively high rate of morbidity after surgical resection remains a current major issue despite the potential of

"cure." Because nonvestibular schwannomas are histologically benign, it must be borne in mind that the goal of the management for patients harboring nonvestibular schwannomas is not to achieve complete resection with some neurologic deficits, but to obtain a good tumor control with preservation of neurologic function for their life span. During the last several decades, stereotactic radiosurgery (SRS) has emerged as a minimally invasive alternative to surgical resection. This article addresses the safety and efficacy of SRS for nonvestibular schwannomas.

THERAPEUTIC OPTIONS

Treatment options include the wait-and-see approach with serial images, microsurgery, and SRS. If patients have asymptomatic tumors, a wait-and-see approach with serial images may be a reasonable treatment option, particularly in older patients or those with comorbidities, because nonvestibular schwannomas are generally slow-growing tumors. At present, there is little

Financial Disclosures: None.
Conflicts of Interest: None.
Department of Neurosurgery, Gamma Knife Center, Komaki City Hospital, 1-20 Jobushi, Komaki, Aichi Prefecture 485-8520, Japan
E-mail address: h-toshi@komakihp.gr.jp

Table 1
Stereotactic radiosurgery series of nonvestibular schwannoma

No. of Patients	Methods	CN (No. of Lesions)	Tumor Volume [Range] (cm³)	Marginal Dose [Range] (Gy)	Follow-Up (mo)	Tumor Control Rate (%)	Improvement of Clinical Symptoms/ Signs (%)	New or Worsening Symptoms (%), No. of Patients
56	GK	V	8.7 (mean) [0.8–33]	13.3 (mean) [10–15]	68 (mean)	93 (crude)	39 (70%)	9 (16%) Facial numbness, 5 Masseter muscle atrophy, 4
37	GK	V	10.3 (mean) [1.2–40.4]	14.2 (mean) [11–16]	54 (mean)	84 (5, 10-y)	14 (40%)	5 (14%) Facial numbness, 3 Facial pain, 3 Corneal ulcer, 1 Abducens palsy, 1
33	GK	V	4.2 (median) [0.5–18.0]	15 (median) [12–20]	72 (mean)	82 (5,10-y)	11 (33%)	3 (9%) Facial sensory loss, 1 Facial pain, 1, Unknown, 1
74	GK	V	5.3 (mean) [0.4–19.9]	16.4 (mean) [12–30]	48.2 (mean)	93 (5-y) 79 (10-y)	8 (11%)	7 (9%) Diplopia, 1 Permanent facial paresthesia, 3 Permanent facial numbness, 2 Transient facial numbness, 1
14	GK	VII	5.5 (mean) [1.0–20.8]	12.9 (mean) [11–16]	31.4 (mean)	100 (crude)	5 (42%)	1 (7%) Facial palsy, 1
11	GK	VII	0.9 (mean) [0.05–2.3]	13 (mean) [10–16]	39 (mean)	91 (crude)	3 (38%)[a]	None
34	GK	JF	4.2 (median) [0.6–10.4]	14 (median) [12–18]	84 (median)	97 (5-y) 94 (10-y)	(20%)[b]	1 (3%) NA

17	GK	JF	5.9 (mean) [1.1–12.3]	13 (mean) [10–16]	64 (mean)	100 (crude)	6 (35%)	1 (6%) Transient hoarseness, 1
49	Linac	III (2), V (25), VII (2), XII (1), JF (18), RS (1)	4.8 (median) [0.35–15.1]	12.5 (median) [10–15]	37 (median)	83 (5-y)	11 (26%)	5 (12%) Facial numbness, 2; Mild anesthesia dolorosa, 1; Facial palsy, 1; Transient diplopia, 1
40	CK (single- and multisession)	IV (1), V (18), VII (6), X (5), XII (2), JF (8), CS (2)	3.2 (median) [0.1–23.7]	18 (median) [15–33]; 17.5 (1 fraction); 20 (2 fractions); 18 (3 fractions)	29 (median)	96 (3-y)	5 (14%)	2 (5%) Jaw weakness and facial numbness, 1; Facial weakness and tinnitus, 1
36	GK	III (1), IV (1), V (25), VI (2), VII (6), IX (1), XII (3), JF (2)	2.9 (median) [0.07–8.8]	13.5 (median) [9.3–20]	37 (median)	91 (2-y); 78 (5-y)	21 (64%)	4 (12%) Facial paresthesia, 2; Lower and upper extremity tremors, paresthesia, slurred speech, tongue deviation and speech, Drooling, 1; Died, 1

Abbreviations: CK, cyberknife; CN, cranial nerve; CS, cavernous sinus; GK, gamma knife; JF, jugular foramen; NA, no data available; RS, retrostyloid.

[a] 3 of 8 patients who had facial palsy before treatment.
[b] 22 of 105 ipsilateral motor cranial nerves including IX,X,XI and XII.

Data from Refs.[3–13]

information about long-term natural history of non-vestibular schwannomas because of their rarity. If considering that any intervention after tumor growth may increase the risk of complications, earlier intervention is advisable to reduce complications. Microsurgery was a common treatment before the advent of SRS. Complete resection is an ideal treatment, but is not so easily achievable without any complications. Although recently skull-base surgery has contributed to an increased rate of complete resection, there is no doubt that this is one of the most invasive treatments. SRS is a less invasive treatment option for small to medium-sized nonvestibular schwannomas, with good tumor control as well as a lower complication rate.

CLINICAL OUTCOMES

Contemporary series of radiosurgery for nonvestibular schwannomas are shown in **Table 1**.

Trigeminal Schwannomas

At the author's institution, 37 trigeminal schwannoma patients treated with gamma-knife radiosurgery (GKRS) were evaluated.[4] Of these patients, 23 (38%) had solid tumors and 14 (62%) had tumors with a cystic component. Seventeen tumors (46%) were located predominantly in the middle fossa, 12 (32%) were located predominantly in the posterior fossa, and 8 (22%) were dumbbell-shaped lesions involving the middle and posterior fossa. Twenty patients (54%) underwent GKRS as

an initial treatment. Mean tumor volume was 10 cm^3 and mean marginal dose was 14 Gy. During the mean follow-up period of 54 months (range 12–140 months), 4 patients (11%) achieved complete remission, 20 (54%) had partial remission, 8 (22%) had stable tumors, and 5 (14%) developed tumor progression or uncontrollable facial pain requiring surgical resection. With a Kaplan-Meier method, actuarial progression-free survival was 84% at both 5 and 10 years. Excluding 2 cases whereby only partial treatment was given because of large tumor volume, these rates increased to 91%. A typical case of trigeminal schwannoma is shown in **Fig. 1**. Of 35 patients who had neurologic symptoms before GKRS, 14 (40%) exhibited some degree of improvement in their symptoms, including reduced facial numbness in 12 patients, resolved facial pain in 6, and resolved diplopia in 4. On the other hand, 5 patients (14%) had newly developed or worsened preexisting symptoms, including facial numbness in 3, facial pain in 3, corneal ulcer in 1, and abducens palsy in 1. Among these patients, 4 developed neurologic deterioration caused by tumor progression while 1 patient developed facial numbness despite tumor regression, thought to be due to adverse radiation effects. Similarly, Kano and colleagues[5] reported the results of GKRS in 33 patients with trigeminal schwannomas. The median radiosurgery target volume was 4.2 cm^3 and the median marginal dose was 15 Gy. At a mean follow-up period of 6 years (range 7–148 months), actuarial progression-free survival was 82% at both 5 and

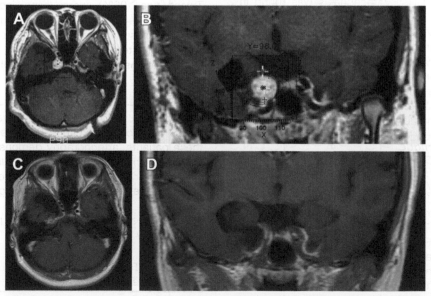

Fig. 1. Axial and coronal T1-weighted magnetic resonance images with gadolinium enhancement, showing a trigeminal schwannoma at the time of gamma-knife radiosurgery (A, B) and 17 years after treatment (C, D).

10 years. Eleven of 33 patients (33%) achieved improved symptoms or signs, and 3 (9%) developed neurologic deterioration.

Facial Schwannomas

In a study by the author's group,[7] 14 patients harboring facial schwannomas were treated using GKRS with a mean marginal dose of 12.9 Gy. The tumor volume varied from 0.98 to 20.8 cm^3 with a mean volume of 5.5 cm^3. The majority of patients presented with facial palsy (11 of 14 patients, 79%) and/or hearing disturbance (9 of 14 patients, 64%). Facial function at the time of GKRS demonstrated a House-Brackmann (HB) Grade I in 3 patients, Grade II in 5, Grade III in 3, and Grade IV in 3. Similarly, hearing function based on Gardner-Robertson classification revealed Class I in 5 patients, Class II in 4, and Class IV in 5. The other symptoms before GKRS included facial hypesthesia in 2 patients, vertigo in 2, dysgeusia in 1, and increased lacrimation in 1. Tumors were located in the geniculate ganglion (2 patients), geniculate ganglion extending into middle fossa (7 patients), cerebellopontine angle (3 patients), and internal meatus (2 patients). Five patients underwent GKRS as the initial treatment, diagnosed on the basis of their common clinical symptoms of facial palsy and the typical radiologic findings showing that the tumor was located in the geniculate ganglion extending into middle cranial fossa. During a mean follow-up period of 31 months, no patient experienced treatment failure. A typical case of facial schwannoma is illustrated in **Fig. 2**.

Facial palsy improved in 5 patients, was stable in 6, and worsened in 1. Two patients retained normal facial function. In 1 patient, facial palsy worsened from an HB Grade I to Grade III within 24 hours after treatment, and did not recover. Hearing function generally remained unchanged. No adverse radiation effect other than worsened facial palsy in 1 patient was found. Litre and colleagues[8] reported the results of 11 facial schwannoma patients who were treated with GKRS. Ten of 11 patients achieved good tumor control with a mean follow-up period of 39 months, demonstrating a crude tumor control rate of 91%. One patient alone developed cyst formation requiring surgical resection. Three of 8 patients who had facial palsy of HB Grade II to IV before treatment achieved improvement of facial nerve function, and no patient had worsening of facial function.

Jugular Foramen Schwannomas

Thirty-three patients harboring jugular foramen schwannomas were treated with GKRS at the author's institution, among whom 16 underwent GKRS as the initial treatment. The mean marginal dose was 13.3 Gy and the mean tumor volume was 8.7 cm^3. During a mean follow-up period of 60 months, 31 of 33 patients (94%) achieved good tumor control, whereas only 2 patients developed tumor progression. A typical case of jugular foramen schwannoma is shown in **Fig. 3**. The most common improved symptom after GKRS was swallowing disturbance in 10 of 13 patients (77%) and hoarseness in 13 of 18 patients (76%).

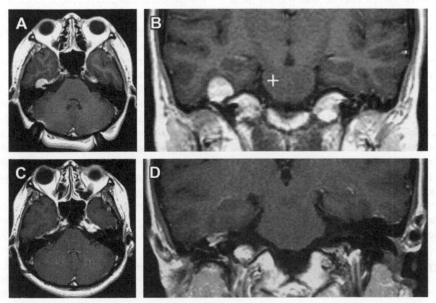

Fig. 2. Axial and coronal T1-weighted magnetic resonance images with gadolinium enhancement, showing a facial schwannoma at the time of gamma-knife radiosurgery (A, B) and 5 years after treatment (C, D).

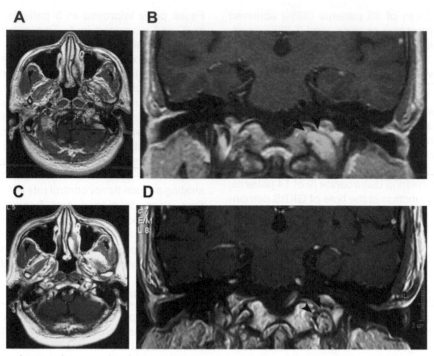

Fig. 3. Axial and coronal T1-weighted magnetic resonance images with gadolinium enhancement, showing a jugular foramen schwannoma (*arrowheads*) at the time of gamma knife radiosurgery (*A, B*) and 10 years after treatment (*C, D*).

There was no neurologic deterioration, other than 2 patients who had worsened hearing function. Martin and colleagues[9] documented the results of 34 patients with jugular foramen schwannoma with 35 tumors, 1 of whom had bilateral tumors. Among these patients, 22 had prior microsurgical resection. Median tumor volume was 4.2 cm³ and median marginal dose was 14 Gy. During a mean follow-up period of 83 months, 17 patients achieved tumor remission, 16 had stable tumors, and 2 developed tumor progression. The actuarial 5- and 10-year progression-free survivals were 97% and 94%, respectively. Regarding functional outcomes, preexisting cranial neuropathies improved in 20% of the affected cranial nerves, remained stable in 77%, and worsened in 2%. One patient developed functional deterioration because of tumor progression. The investigators found that 138 of 140 (98%) motor cranial nerves remained intact or improved after GKRS. If limited to patients who had no prior surgical resection, 47% of affected cranial nerves showed improvement at a median period of 16 months after treatment.

COMPLICATIONS AND CONCERNS

To compare the results between SRS and microsurgery, current microsurgical series of nonvestibular schwannomas are shown in **Table 2**. In comparisons of these series, complication rates after SRS are much lower than those after microsurgery. In cases of trigeminal schwannomas, facial hypesthesia is the most common adverse radiation effect. The rate of newly developed or worsened symptoms after SRS varied from 9% to 16% with a mean marginal dose of 13 to 16 Gy. As long as the tumor does not grow, newly developed or worsened neurologic deficits, other than trigeminal nerve injury, as adverse radiation effects are extremely rare. Some patients develop facial pain, probably caused by tumor adhesion from irradiation, or a type of paresthesia caused by radiation injury to the trigeminal nerve. According to published articles,[3–6] the tumor control rate of trigeminal schwannomas treated with SRS tends to be slightly worse than rates of the other schwannomas including vestibular, facial, or jugular foramen schwannomas. Treatment failure is likely to occur with cyst formation or refractory facial pain requiring tumor resection. Regarding outcomes of microsurgery for trigeminal schwannomas in comparison with radiosurgical series cranial nerve injuries other than fifth-nerve injury are more common, but recent advanced skull-base techniques seem to contribute to improved outcomes and a high rate of complete tumor resection for trigeminal schwannoma, particularly if predominantly located in the middle fossa. Nevertheless,

Table 2
Results of microsurgery for nonvestibular schwannomas

CN	No. of Patients	Approach	Follow-Up Period (mo)	Resection	Tumor Control Rate (%)	Tumor Recurrence Rate (%)	Morbidity	Mortality Rate (%)
V	58	Subtemporal combined extradural/intradural, 18 Subtemporal extradural, 8 Subtemporal orbitozygomatic, 15 Retrosigmoid, 12 Staged (retromastoid/subtemporal), 3 Combined presigmoid-subtemporal, 2	62 (mean)	CTR, 48 PTR, 10	NA 76 (CTR) 24 (PTR)	NA 5 (re-operation)	III deficit, 2 (transient) IV deficit, 2 (persistent), 2 (transient) Corneal ulceration, 5 (persistent) VII deficit, 2 (persistent), 3 (transient) Meningitis, 5 CSF leakage, 3 Chest infection, 4	2
V	42	Frontotemporal transsylvian, 3 Subtemporal intradural, 5 Retrosigmoid, 8 Subtemporal transtentorial, 4 Orbitozygomatic infratemporal, 6 Zygomatic infratemporal, 8 Frontotemporal transsylvian/zygomatic infratemporal, 3 Presigmoid transpetrosal transtentorial, 5	6–144	CTR, 28 NTR, 10 PTR, 4[b]	88[a] (crude)	12	III deficit, 2 V deficit, 5 VI deficit, 1 VII deficit, 1 VIII deficit, 4	0

(continued on next page)

Table 2
(continued)

CN	No. of Patients	Approach	Follow-Up Period (mo)	Resection	Tumor Control Rate (%)	Tumor Recurrence Rate (%)	Morbidity	Mortality Rate (%)
V	57	Frontotemporal, 4 Subtemporal, 6 Lateral suboccipital, 2 Orbitozygomatic, 3 Zygomatic infratemporal, 2 Orbitozygomatic infratemporal, 1 Anterior transpetrosal, 29 Zygomatic transpetrosal, 7 Supraorbital, 1 Transzygomatic, 2	4.9 (mean)	CTR, 46 NTR, 3 PTR, 7 Biopsy, 1	98 (crude)	2	Total ophthalmoplegia, 2 III deficit, 1 (persistent), 2 (transient) IV deficit, 1 (persistent), 2 (transient) V deficit, 23 VI deficit, 4 (persistent), 5 (transient) VII deficit, 2 (persistent) Temporal lobe contusion, 2 CSF leakage, 2 Peripheral neuropathy of lower extremity, 1	0
VII	33 (36 surgeries)	Translabyrinthine, 17 Retrosigmoid, 6 Combined transmastoid/middle cranial fossa, 3 Combined transmastoid/transparotid, 3 Transmastoid, 2 Middle cranial fossa, 1 Transotic, 1	NA	CTR, 21 STR, 4 Other, 11	NA	NA	Sacrificed VII nerve, 21 Wound infection and CSF leak, 1 Intractable vertigo, 1 Significant headache, 1 External auditory canal stenosis, 1 XII deficit, 1	0
VII	53	Translabyrinthine, 55% Transmastoid, 11% Combined transmastoid/middle cranial fossa, 11% Middle cranial fossa, 9% Retrosigmoid, 9% Combined translabyrinthine/middle cranial fossa, 4%	NA	CTR, 45 STR, 8	100	NA	Sacrificed VII nerve, 36	0

		Surgical approach	Follow-up	Resection	Tumor control (%)	Recurrence	Complications	Mortality
JF	53	Retrosigmoid, 12 Extreme lateral infrajugular transtubercular, 23 Extreme lateral infrajugular transtubercular/transjugular, 15 Extreme lateral infrajugular transtubercular/transjugular/high cervical, 3	101 (mean)	CTR, 48 Other, 4	94 (crude)	6	VII deficit, 2 VIII deficit, 4 IX & X deficit, 14 XI deficit, 6 XII deficit, 7	0
JF	22 (25 surgeries)	Infratemporal fossa, 3 Transcochlear/transjugular, 1 Petrooccipital transsigmoid, 13 Petrooccipital transsigmoid/translabyrinthine, 1 Petrooccipital transsigmoid/transotic, 2 Translabyrinthine, 1 Translabyrinthine/transsigmoid-transjugular, 1 Transcervical/subtotal petrosectomy, 2 Transcervical, 1	NA	CTR, 21 STR, 1 Waiting for the second stage, 1	100	0	Lower cranial nerve deficit, 11 VII deficit, 2 (persistent), 2 (transient) VIII deficit, 10 CSF leakage and meningitis, 1 Subcutaneous CSF collection, 2	0
JF	16	Juxtacondylar	79 (mean)	CTR, 13 STR, 3	100	0	Aspiration pneumonia, 1 CSF leakage, 1 Transient swallowing disturbance, 4	0
JF	15	Lateral suboccipital, 12 Combined transjugular and suboccipital, 2 Infralabyrinthine, 1	84 (median)	NTR, 10 STR, 5	70 (5-y)	53	IX, X deficit, 9 (postoperative), 3 (final)	0

(continued on next page)

Table 2
(continued)

CN	No. of Patients	Approach	Follow-Up Period (mo)	Resection	Tumor Control Rate (%)	Tumor Recurrence Rate (%)	Morbidity	Mortality Rate (%)
JF	81	NA	NA	CTR, 54 NTR, 23 STR, 1	91 (crude)	9	VI deficit, 1 (persistent), 0 (transient) VII deficit, 3 (persistent), 6 (transient) VIII deficit, 5 (persistent), 4 (transient) IX/X deficit, 16 (persistent), 23 (transient) XI deficit, 7 (persistent), 9 (transient) XII deficit, 8 (persistent), 9 (transient) CSF leakage, 3 Postoperative ICH, 2	0
III 1 IV 2 V 24 VI 1 VII 3 JF 7 X 2 XII 3		Orbitozygomatic Retrosigmoid Far-lateral Transpetrosal Far-lateral/transpetrosal Retrosigmoid/transpetrosal Retrosigmoid/orbitozygomatic Others	45 (mean)	NA	97[a] (crude)	3[a]	CSF leakage, 5 Hydrocephalus, 1 Postoperative ICH, 1 IV deficit, 1 V deficit, 1 VIII deficit, 4 Dysphagia with tracheostomy and PEG, 1	0

Abbreviations: CN, cranial nerve; CSF, cerebrospinal fluid; CTR, complete tumor resection; ICH, intracerebral hematoma; JF, jugular foramen; NA, not available; NTR, near total resection (>95%); PEG, percutaneous endoscopic gastrostomy; PTR, partial tumor resection; STR, subtotal resection (>90%).
[a] Limited results of 24 trigeminal and 7 jugular foramen schwannomas.
[b] All patients were followed by radiosurgery.
Data from Refs.[14–24]

complete resection still remains challenging for most neurosurgeons because of the rarity of this tumor. In cases of facial schwannomas, Kida and colleagues[7] reported that 1 patient developed persistent facial palsy of HB Grade II, whereas Litre and colleagues[8] did not experience any patients who developed facial palsy. These small series provide important information that SRS for facial schwannomas is much safer than surgical resection, although the number of patients is somewhat limited. Surprisingly, hearing deterioration is unlikely to occur as an adverse radiation effect. McRackan and colleagues[18] described the results of 53 patients with a facial schwannoma who underwent surgical resection (total resection 45, subtotal resection 8). Thirty-three patients (52%) had normal facial function of HB Grade I before treatment. Facial nerve was sacrificed in 36 of 53 patients (68%) at the time of surgery. At 1 year after surgical resection, only 7 patients retained HB Grade I. Subtotal resection was found to be a significant factor in relation to postoperative facial preservation of HB Grade III or better, indicating that total resection without facial nerve injury is almost infeasible. McMonagle and colleagues[17] also reported the difficulty of preserving facial function in 33 patients with facial schwannoma who underwent surgical resection. In this series 21 nerve reconstructions were eventually required. The investigators concluded that surgical intervention for facial schwannomas should be indicated when facial function deteriorates to an HB Grade IV. At present, SRS is definitely superior to microsurgery with regard to facial nerve preservation. Similarly, in cases of jugular foramen schwannomas, an incidence of newly developed or worsened neurologic deficits after SRS is considered rare. In the author's experience, no patient developed deterioration of ninth or tenth cranial nerve after SRS. On the contrary, more than 70% of patients who had swallowing disturbance and/or hoarseness before treatment showed improvement after SRS. Compared with other symptomatic schwannomas, it seems that patients with jugular foramen schwannomas treated with SRS as the initial treatment are more likely to improve their symptoms. In other words, a high rate of symptomatic improvement could be expected if a ninth or tenth cranial nerve were not injured at the time of tumor resection. On the other hand, microsurgery still has a relatively high risk of complications, even with recent various skull-base techniques in experienced hands. According to microsurgical series of 22 patients with jugular foramen schwannomas reported by Sanna and colleagues,[20] a half of the patients had worsened ninth and tenth cranial nerve function postoperatively. Moreover, Sedney and colleagues[23]

documented that a conservative operative technique of near total resection significantly decreased postoperative permanent ninth and tenth cranial nerve deficits in comparison with a radical gross total resection. Consequently, their surgical strategy for jugular foramen schwannomas was changed from a total resection to a near total resection, to retain neurologic function. When comparing functional outcomes between SRS and microsurgery, SRS promises to be a reasonable alternative to surgical resection in patients harboring jugular foramen schwannomas, as long as the tumor does not compress the brainstem severely.

Regarding treatment dose, as shown in **Table 1**, 13 to 14 Gy to the tumor margin appears to be an optimum dose to achieve both long-term safety and good tumor control for nonvestibular schwannomas. Such a dose level makes sense if extrapolated from the author's experience that vestibular schwannomas have been safely and effectively treated at a marginal dose of 12 to 13 Gy.[25]

SUMMARY

SRS is a safe and effective treatment for patients with small to medium-sized nonvestibular schwannomas. Until now microsurgery has been a common treatment option for nonvestibular schwannomas but, even with recent refinement of microsurgical techniques, it is unable to avoid the risk of complications such as cranial nerve injury, cerebrospinal fluid leakage, or infection. Accordingly, SRS can be a reasonable alternative to surgical resection not only as adjuvant treatment but also as the initial treatment. When the tumor is relatively large (eg, severely compressing the brainstem), it should be first removed with microsurgery. However, complete resection is not necessarily required if cranial nerve injury is strongly predicted. One should keep in mind that the residual tumor can be safely treated with SRS. At this stage, in cases of facial schwannomas or jugular foramen schwannomas, SRS seems to be superior to microsurgery with respect to preservation of cranial nerve function. However, because of the rarity of nonvestibular schwannomas, there is little information about long-term outcomes of SRS at present. It is therefore necessary to collect further long-term follow-up data to clarify the safety and efficacy of SRS for nonvestibular schwannomas.

REFERENCES

1. Mabanta SR, Buatti JM, Friedman WA, et al. Linear accelerator radiosurgery for nonacoustic schwannomas. Int J Radiat Oncol Biol Phys 1999;43:545–8.

2. Pollock BE, Foote RL, Stafford SL. Stereotactic radiosurgery: the preferred management for patients with nonvestibular schwannomas? Int J Radiat Oncol Biol Phys 2002;52:1002–7.

3. Pan L, Wang EM, Zhang N, et al. Long-term results of Leksell gamma knife surgery for trigeminal schwannomas. J Neurosurg 2005;102(Suppl): 220–4.

4. Hasegawa T, Kida Y, Yoshimoto M, et al. Trigeminal schwannomas: results of gamma knife surgery in 37 cases. J Neurosurg 2007;106:18–23.

5. Kano H, Niranjan A, Kondziolka D, et al. Stereotactic radiosurgery for trigeminal schwannomas: tumor control and functional preservation. J Neurosurg 2009;110:553–8.

6. Yianni J, Dinca EB, Rowe J, et al. Stereotactic radiosurgery for trigeminal schwannomas. Acta Neurochir 2012;154:277–83.

7. Kida Y, Yoshimoto M, Hasegawa T. Radiosurgery for facial schwannoma. J Neurosurg 2007;106:24–9.

8. Litre CF, Goug GP, Tamura M, et al. Gamma knife surgery for facial nerve schwannomas. Neurosurgery 2007;60:853–9.

9. Martin JJ, Kondziolka D, Flickinger JC, et al. Cranial nerve preservation and outcomes after stereotactic radiosurgery for jugular foramen schwannomas. Neurosurgery 2007;61:76–81.

10. Peker S, Sengöz M, Kılıç T, et al. Gamma knife radiosurgery for jugular foramen schwannomas. Neurosurg Rev 2012;35:549–53.

11. Kimball MM, Foote KD, Bova FJ, et al. Linear accelerator radiosurgery for nonvestibular schwannomas. Neurosurgery 2011;68:974–84.

12. Choi CY, Soltys SG, Gibbs IC, et al. Stereotactic radiosurgery of cranial nonvestibular schwannomas: results of single- and multisession radiosurgery. Neurosurgery 2011;68:1200–8.

13. Elsharkawy M, Xu Z, Schlesinger D, et al. Gamma knife surgery for nonvestibular schwannomas: radiological and clinical outcomes. J Neurosurg 2012; 116:66–72.

14. Sharma BS, Ahmad FU, Chandra PS, et al. Trigeminal schwannomas: experience with 68 cases. J Clin Neurosci 2008;15:738–43.

15. Zhang L, Yang Y, Xu S, et al. Trigeminal schwannomas: a report of 42 cases and review of the relevant surgical approaches. Clin Neurol Neurosurg 2009; 111:261–9.

16. Fukaya R, Yoshida K, Ohira T, et al. Trigeminal schwannomas: experience with 57 cases and a review of the literature. Neurosurg Rev 2011;34:159–71.

17. McMonagle B, Al-Sanosi A, Croxson G, et al. Facial schwannoma: results of a large case series and review. J Laryngol Otol 2008;122:1139–50.

18. McRackan TR, Rivas A, Wanna GB, et al. Facial nerve outcomes in facial nerve schwannomas. Otol Neurotol 2012;33:78–82.

19. Bulsara KR, Sameshima T, Friedman AH, et al. Microsurgical management of 53 jugular foramen schwannomas: lessons learned incorporated into a modified grading system. J Neurosurg 2008;109: 794–803.

20. Sanna M, Bacciu A, Falcioni M, et al. Surgical management of jugular foramen schwannomas with hearing and facial nerve function preservation: a series of 23 cases and review of the literature. Laryngoscope 2006;116:2191–204.

21. Chibbaro S, Mirone G, Makiese O, et al. Dumbbell-shaped jugular foramen schwannomas: surgical management, outcome and complications on a series of 16 patients. Neurosurg Rev 2009;32:151–9.

22. Fukuda M, Oishi M, Saito A, et al. Long-term outcomes after surgical treatment of jugular foramen schwannoma. Skull Base 2009;19:401–8.

23. Sedney CL, Nonaka Y, Bulsara KR, et al. Microsurgical management of jugular foramen schwannomas. Neurosurgery 2013;72(1):42–6. http://dx.doi.org/10. 1227//NEU.0b013e3182770e74 [discussion: 46].

24. Salvi-Abbasi S, Bambakidis NC, Zabramski JM, et al. Nonvestibular schwannomas: an evaluation of functional outcome after radiosurgical and microsurgical management. Acta Neurochir 2010;152:35–46.

25. Hasegawa T, Kida Y, Kato T, et al. Long-term safety and efficacy of stereotactic radiosurgery for vestibular schwannomas: evaluation of 440 patients more than 10 years after treatment with gamma knife surgery. J Neurosurg 2013;118(3):557–65. http://dx. doi.org/10.3171/2012.10.JNS12523.

Multi-Session Radiosurgery of Benign Intracranial Tumors

Jacky T. Yeung, MD, Syed Aftab Karim, MD,
Steven D. Chang, MD*

KEYWORDS

• Radiosurgery • Benign • Intracranial tumors • Tumors

KEY POINTS

• Multi-session stereotactic radiosurgery (SRS) may play a key radiosurgical role in the treatment of tumors adjacent to sensitive neurologic structures.
• Multi-session SRS enables a high dose per fraction to be delivered because the rapid dose falloff allows for sparing of critical structures.
• Initial experiences with multi-session SRS have demonstrated efficacy and safety in the treatment of benign intracranial tumors, including meningiomas, vestibular schwannomas, and pituitary adenomas.

INTRODUCTION: NATURE OF THE PROBLEM

Benign intracranial tumors, commonly including meningiomas, vestibular schwannomas, and pituitary adenomas, present a challenge to neuro-oncologists and neurosurgeons. The management of these tumors includes surgical resection, radiotherapy, and, at times, observation. Although surgical resection has been the gold standard treatment of large and clinically symptomatic lesions, the decision to resect these slow-growing tumors may be hindered by patients' unwillingness to endure the invasive nature of the procedures for a benign lesion. Some cases of benign intracranial tumors may not be amenable to surgical resection when they are in unfavorable anatomic locations and involve critical structures. Despite the generally benign nature of the aforementioned tumors, recurrences do occur and present a further clinical dilemma for the clinician and patients.

Stereotactic radiosurgery (SRS) is a combination of stereotactic localization techniques invented in neurosurgery and radiation physics used to deliver concentrated energy, in the form of X rays, gamma rays, and protons, to an image-guided anatomic location. This therapeutic modality allows the clinician to deliver a destructive dose of radiation to an intended target while minimizing damage to adjacent structures. Initially conceived by Lars Leksell[1] of the Karolinska Institute in Stockholm in the 1950s, SRS has dramatically improved in patient outcomes with the advances in neuroimaging and dose-planning algorithms. SRS is now a treatment option for a plethora of intracranial pathologic conditions, ranging from brain tumors to arteriovenous malformations. Particularly, benign intracranial tumors are good candidates for SRS because of their slow growth rates and well-circumscribed borders. Advanced magnetic resonance imaging (MRI) can, in most cases, capture the entirety of these benign tumors and delineate tumor and normal structures. Benign tumors are considered to behave like late-responding normal tissue[2] and may respond better to higher doses per fraction. This technique for radiation delivery may result in greater tumor shrinkage than conventional irradiation techniques.[3]

Disclosures: The authors have nothing to disclose.
Department of Neurosurgery, Stanford University School of Medicine, 300 Pasteur Drive, Room R-225, Stanford, CA 94305, USA
* Corresponding author.
E-mail address: sdchang@stanford.edu

neurosurgery.theclinics.com

At Stanford University, the authors used the CyberKnife SRS system with a multi-session schedule to treat benign intracranial tumors. Multi-session SRS enables a high dose per fraction to be delivered and, along with the rapid dose falloff, allows for sparing of critical structures, theoretically, resulting in less radiation-associated toxicity.[4] There may also be increased tumor cytotoxicity from interfraction reoxygenation and reassortment.[4] Multi-sessions also allow for a shorter treatment duration that is more convenient for patients than conventional radiation courses.

SRS is now a commonly used treatment modality for benign intracranial tumors. This article reviews the basic concepts and techniques of multi-session SRS, indications for this technique, and the outcomes from single-session and multi-session SRS using 3 commonly treated benign intracranial tumors (meningiomas, vestibular schwannomas, pituitary adenomas) as points of discussion.

INDICATIONS AND TECHNIQUES
Indications for SRS

Patients with newly presenting or recurrent benign intracranial neoplasms, determined based on imaging, biopsy, and history, may be given choices for surgical resection, SRS, and observation. Those patients who may benefit maximally from multi-session SRS often have the following characteristics:

1. Radiographic evidence of tumor progression after prior treatment
2. Symptomatic, untreated lesions with unfavorable locations for open surgery
3. Symptomatic lesions in patients who were poor surgical candidates because of advanced age or medical comorbidities
4. Patients choose to deny observation but refuse open surgery

Large benign tumors or tumors adjacent to sensitive critical neurologic structures, such as the optic nerve, may benefit from multi-session radiosurgery over single-session techniques.

Radiosurgical Technique

The CyberKnife Robotic Radiosurgical System (Accuray, Inc, Sunnyvale, California) was used to deliver the radiosurgical treatments. A high-resolution, thin-slice (1.25 mm) computed tomogram (CT) was obtained using a GE Light Speed 8i or 16i Scanner (Milwaukee, Wisconsin) after the administration of 125 mL of Omnipaque

intravenous contrast (iohexol, 350 mg I/mL; Nycomed, Inc, GE Healthcare, Princeton, New Jersey). A stereotactic MRI scan was obtained and fused to the stereotactic CT scan to improve the target identification.

SRS is a joined effort among the neurosurgeon, radiation oncologist, and radiation physicist during the processes of tumor delineation, dose selection, and planning. The gross tumor volume of most benign intracranial neoplasms is defined as the residual or recurrent enhanced (if contrast enhancing) tumor seen on imaging. The radiosurgical dose is prescribed to cover the gross tumor volume with no additional margin. The treatment plan is created using the CyberKnife nonisocentric inverse treatment planning software. Once image-guided registration is performed, radiosurgery is administered to awake and usually unanesthetized patients. At the authors' institution, patients have historically been given 4 mg of dexamethasone as well as antinausea medications as needed either before or after each treatment.

The quality of treatment plans is assessed by evaluating target coverage, dose heterogeneity, and conformity. Digitally reconstructed radiograms were computationally synthesized to allow near real-time patient tracking throughout radiosurgery. For multi-session treatments, the typical interfraction time interval was 24 hours.

Radiosurgical Dosage

SRS is a technique built largely on published center-specific experiences. Therefore, there is no strict dose selection for a specific pathological condition. Rather, it takes into account several patient- and center-specific factors. At Stanford University, the initial dose selection for multi-session radiosurgery was based on the following:

1. Extrapolation from the published single-fraction radiosurgery experience
2. A calculated biologic effective dose (BED) based on conventionally fractionated radiotherapy
3. A previous experience with fractionated frame-based radiosurgery for similar tumors[4]

Afterward, the dose and fractionation decision for each patient depends on tumor volume, location, patient age, tumor histology, proximity to crucial neural structures, and history of irradiation.

A BED can be estimated from the following formula[5]:

$$BED = nd(1 + d/(\alpha \times \beta))$$

where n is the number of fractions (sessions), d is the dose per fraction (session), α/β is the α-to-β ratio, an estimate of the radiation sensitivity. An α-to-β ratio of 3 is accepted to represent the value that estimates the sensitivity of late-responding tissue, whereas a value of 10 corresponds to early responding tissue. Benign intracranial tumors are considered to be late-responding tissue because of slow proliferation, so a lower α-to-β ratio is used in most cases. The lower and upper limits of the α-to-β ratio estimates of the World Health Organization (WHO) grade I meningioma have been calculated to be 2.7 to 3.9.[2] The α-to-β ratio used for WHO grade II meningioma at Stanford University has been 4, which is equivalent to a median single-session dose of 18 Gy.[6] In vestibular schwannoma, the radiation dose ranges from 12 Gy for maximal hearing preservation in patients with smaller tumors to 13 Gy to the tumor margin for patients with deafness related to prior resection.[7] For functional pituitary adenomas, studies using GammaKnife radiosurgery have reported using marginal doses ranging from 15 Gy to 34 Gy in one session.[8] Pollock and colleagues[9] have reported the use of a median marginal dose of 20 Gy with satisfactory results.

Multi-session SRS is routinely performed on an outpatient basis with an interfraction time of approximately 24 hours. When minimal toxicity is observed with multi-session radiosurgery, the prescribed radiobiologic dose can be gradually escalated. Dose escalation can be accomplished by either an increase in the dose per session or by a decrease in the number of sessions.

CLINICAL OUTCOMES
Meningiomas

Meningiomas are the most common nonglial primary intracranial tumors in adults.[10] The main goal of management for these tumors is to minimize mass-induced symptoms. Small, asymptomatic lesions can have variable growth rates and can be observed with serial imaging.[11] Easily accessible meningiomas can be easily treated with surgical resection. However, those in more eloquent locations, such as the skull base, and those that surround important neurovascular structures are less amenable to complete resection without severe morbidities. It has been estimated that 20% to 30% of meningioma cases are not amenable to complete surgical resection.[12,13] For such reasons, SRS has become an attractive primary or adjuvant mode of treatment of meningiomas.

Local control rates following SRS of benign meningiomas were reported to range from 86% to 100% at 5 years and 83% to 95% at 10 years.[14–17] Using historical control, Pollock

and colleagues[18] found that primary SRS for small- and medium-sized meningiomas had equivalent tumor control rates for SRS compared with Simpson grade I resection at 3 and 7 years. For less complete resections (Simpson grade II–IV), SRS provided better progression-free survival (PFS) at 3 and 7 years.[18] The comparison of SRS and open surgery remains indirect because no such parallel studies exist and retrospective studies of this nature inherently carries substantial selection bias. However, the data thus far suggest that SRS as the primary treatment modality was somewhat comparable with open resection and without the invasiveness.

For skull-base meningiomas, which represent anatomic challenges for resection, Zachenhofer and colleagues[19] reported no radiologic or symptomatic progression at late follow-up for the SRS-alone group and equivalent rates of neurologic improvement between the surgical and nonsurgical groups. In a series of 255 cases of skull-base meningiomas treated with GammaKnife SRS, Starke and colleagues[20] reported actuarial PFS rates at 3, 5, and 10 years to be 99%, 96%, and 79%, respectively. Their data suggest that SRS can offer a good tumor control and neurologic preservation in patients with skull-base meningiomas, including those situated at the cerebellopontine angle, parasellar, or petroclival location.[20]

Cavernous sinus meningiomas are a distinct variety with SRS being a favorable treatment option because of its anatomic location. The 5-year actuarial PFS is reported to be between 93% and 100%.[21,22] In a series by Pollock and colleagues,[22] 49 patients with dural-based masses of the cavernous sinus presumed to be meningiomas (mean tumor volume of 10.2 mL) were treated with a mean tumor margin dose of 15.9 Gy. No tumor enlargement was reported after SRS.[22] Twelve of 38 patients (26%) with preexisting diplopia or facial symptoms improved in cranial nerve function.[22] Although more data are needed to assert the efficacy of SRS as the primary treatment of cavernous sinus meningiomas, SRS can be an effective option for these tumors after the risk of open surgery is discussed with patients. Open surgery may be more useful in cases with a symptomatic mass effect or atypical imaging features that may suggest alternative or malignant tumor characteristics to confirm the histologic diagnosis.

Although SRS is a reasonable option for the treatment of meningiomas, limitations exist in the management of higher-grade tumors. In a review by Kondziolka and colleagues[23] of 972 patients over an 18-year interval, even though the 10-year actuarial tumor control rate for WHO grade I tumors was 87%, the 5-year actuarial tumor control rates for grades II and III tumors were only approximately 30% and 10%, respectively. The risk of intracranial tumor recurrence increased approximately 4 times with increasing WHO grade.[23] The decision to use SRS as a sole primary treatment of seemingly benign meningiomas may, therefore, be better guided by detailed imaging and available histology of the tumors when available.

At the authors' institution, small meningiomas that are not adjacent to critical or sensitive neurologic structures are typically treated with single-session radiosurgery. Multi-session radiosurgery for meningiomas is typically reserved for larger meningiomas (greater than 3 cm), meningiomas located in parasagittal locations where the risk of edema has been shown to be substantially higher than other meningiomas,[24] or for meningiomas located next to the optic or cochlear nerves.

VESTIBULAR SCHWANNOMAS

There is still debate on the management of small- to medium-sized vestibular schwannoma (VS). Several retrospective case-control series have found radiosurgery to provide superior improved facial nerve outcomes and hearing-preservation rates.[25–27] Because of the more conformal dose planning and lower radiation dose prescription, the risk of facial weakness or numbness has dramatically decreased over time.[28]

Because of the nature of VS and its close proximity to critical cranial nerves in the cerebellopontine angle, morbidities from SRS treatment remain high, with some initial radiosurgery series reporting hearing-preservation rates that ranged from 51% to 60% with significant rates of facial weakness and numbness.[29–31] At Stanford University, multi-session SRS is used in an attempt to reduce the risk of injury to adjacent critical structures, especially because studies have shown that total radiation dose to the cochlea is a determining factor in hearing preservation.[32,33] The authors have previously reported using staged CyberKnife SRS in 61 patients with a minimum of 36 months of follow-up.[34] Seventy-four percent of patients with serviceable hearing (Gardner-Robinson class 1–2) maintained serviceable hearing at the last follow-up, and no patient with at least some hearing before treatment lost all hearing on the treated side.[34] Twenty-nine of 61 (48%) tumors decreased in size and 31 (50%) of the 61 tumors were stable.[34] Most importantly, no patients developed new trigeminal dysfunction or permanent injury to their facial nerve.[34] A larger, more recent series of patients with VS treated with multi-session radiosurgery showed a hearing preservation rate of 76%, whereas the 3- and 5-year tumor control rates were 99% and 96%, respectively.[35] Although these data may indicate a possible higher chance of hearing preservation of multi-session radiosurgery compared with single-session radiosurgery, no head-to-head comparison between these two techniques has been made.

As with most SRS studies, direct comparisons of either single-session or multi-session SRS with open surgery are lacking. Pollock and colleagues[36] performed a prospective cohort study of 82 patients with unilateral, unoperated VS less than 3 cm undergoing surgical resection (n = 36) or radiosurgery (n = 46). Normal facial movement and preservation of serviceable hearing were more frequent in the radiosurgical group at 3 months (P<.001), 1 year (P<.001), and at the last follow-up examination (P<.01) compared with the surgical resection group.[36] Patients undergoing surgical resection scored lower on physical functioning (P = .006), role-physical (P<.001), energy/fatigue (P = .02), and overall physical component (P = .004) of the Health Status Questionnaire 3 months after surgery.[36] Unlike patients in the surgical resection group, the radiosurgical group had no decline on any component of the Health Status Questionnaire after the procedure.[36] Their results provided initial support for SRS to be superior in preserving cranial nerve functions and having higher functional outcomes compared with surgical resection for patients with small- to moderate-sized VSs.

There is still no consensus on the optimal dosing for the treatment of VS. Kondziolka and colleagues[29] at the University of Pittsburgh reported 162 patients with VS undergoing radiosurgery between 1987 and 1992 using a relatively higher mean dose of 16 Gy and demonstrated a tumor control rate of 98%. Updated results from the same center on VS radiosurgery for patients (n = 216) receiving tumor margin doses of 12 or 13 Gy reported a similar resection-free control rate of 98% at a median follow-up of 5.7 years.[37] Limited by the quality of studies examining optimal dosing, it remains to be determined whether currently prescribed doses for VS radiosurgery (12–13 Gy) can provide the same high rate of tumor control observed when tumor margin doses were higher (14–16 Gy). Assuming an α-to-β ratio of 3, the multi-session standard SRS dose of 18 Gy in 3 sessions used at Stanford for VS corresponds to a biologically equivalent dose of approximately 12 Gy.

Pituitary Adenomas

Pituitary adenomas are categorized as functioning and nonfunctioning subtypes. Functioning adenomas are hormone producing and result in exaggerated endocrine dysfunctions. Otherwise, patients may present with visual defects secondary to mass effect on the optic nerves and chiasm. The goals of management in patients with pituitary adenomas are multifaceted and include biochemical remission in functioning adenomas, preservation of normal pituitary production of other hormones, improvement in visual function, and local tumor control. A stepwise approach is taken in the management of these patients, starting with medical therapy (dopamine agonist for prolactin-secreting adenomas), surgical resection if a tumor is causing significant symptomatic mass effect, and radiotherapy (fractionated or SRS). The decision to undergo medical and surgical therapy often falls onto the endocrinologist and neurosurgeon. The decision to administer SRS or external beam radiation therapy (EBRT) is largely caused by the anatomic characteristics of a tumor. Poorly defined tumors or those in close proximity to the optic apparatus are best treated with EBRT because the margins cannot be well defined in SRS planning. Later, the authors focus on the use of SRS in controlling these tumors and compare its outcomes with those of fractionated radiotherapy.

Dose selection, much like other intracranial pathologic conditions, is based on histology, tumor size, the distance from adjacent normal structures (optic apparatus in the case of pituitary adenomas), and history of prior radiotherapy. For patients with hormone-secreting tumors, the minimum tumor margin dose is generally from 20 to 25 Gy.[38,39] The dose prescribed for nonfunctioning adenomas generally is slightly lower than those that are functional, with a reported mean dose of 18.4 Gy (range 8–25 Gy) by Gopalan and colleagues.[40] When the maximum dose received by the optic apparatus is less than 12 Gy, postradiosurgical visual deficits are reported to be less than 2%.[41] At Stanford University, the authors recognized the restricted radiation tolerance of the anterior visual pathways as a limitation in single-session radiosurgery. The authors reported their experience with multisession CyberKnife radiosurgery for perioptic lesions, which included 19 cases of pituitary adenomas.[42] Two to 5 sessions of SRS to an average tumor volume of 7.7 cm^3 and a cumulative average marginal dose of 20.3 Gy were used.[42] After a mean visual field follow-up of 49 months (range 6–96 months), vision was unchanged in 38 patients, improved in 8 (16%), and worse in 3 (6%).[42] In each instance, visual deterioration attributed to tumor progression was confirmed with imaging.[42] Seemingly, a multi-session SRS approach can result in high rates of tumor control and preserve visual function in perioptic pituitary adenomas.

SRS is an attractive approach for nonfunctional adenomas with a wealth of data supporting its efficacy and safety. Pollock and colleagues[43] performed a retrospective review of 62 patients with nonfunctional adenomas undergoing radiosurgery between 1992 and 2004, of whom 59 (95%) underwent prior tumor resection. The median treatment volume was 4.0 cm^3 (range 0.8–12.9).[43] The median treatment dose to the tumor margin was 16 Gy (range 11–20).[43] The median maximum point dose to the optic apparatus was 9.5 Gy (range 5.0–12.6).[43] At a median follow-up interval of 64 months, the tumor size decreased for 37 patients (60%) and remained unchanged for 23 patients (37%).[43] Two patients (3%) had tumor growth outside the prescribed treatment volume and required additional treatment.[43] Tumor growth control was 95% at 3 and 7 years after radiosurgery.[43] The risk of developing new anterior pituitary deficits at 5 years was 32%. The investigators reported no decline in visual function in any patient.[43] Similarly, the University of Virginia reported a high rate of tumor control and a low rate of neurologic deficits in their series.[44] They reported on 140 consecutive patients with nonfunctioning pituitary macroadenomas treated using Gamma Knife surgery.[44] Thirteen patients were treated with SRS as the primary therapy, and 127 patients had undergone at least 1 open resection before Gamma Knife surgery.[44] The mean maximal dose was 38.6 Gy (range 10–70 Gy), with a mean marginal dose of 18 Gy (range 5–25 Gy).[44] They reported PFS at 2, 5, 8, and 10 years to be 98%, 97%, 91%, and 87%, respectively.[44] In multivariate analysis, they found tumor volume greater than 5 cm^3 (hazard ratio = 5.0, 95% confidence interval [CI] 1.5–17.2, P = .023) to be the only factor predictive of tumor growth.[44] In their follow-up, delayed hypopituitarism occurred in 30.3% of patients.[44] As expected, visual decline was the most common neurologic deficit (12.8%) in their series; but all patients with visual decline had evidence of tumor progression.[44] In these large series, SRS seems to be an effective and safe option for tumor control with reasonable rates of posttreatment pituitary and visual deficits.

SRS has been reported to be a safe and effective treatment of patients with hormone-secreting pituitary adenomas. In patients with medically refractory prolactin (PRL)-producing adenomas or those who are intolerant to dopamine agonist therapy, Tanaka and colleagues[39] reported biochemical remission off medications and clinical improvement in 4 patients (18%), normal serum PRL concentrations and clinical improvement on dopamine agonist therapy in 3 patients (14%), improved symptoms off medications but continued elevated serum PRL levels in 7 patients (32%), and 8 patients (36%) continued to be symptomatic with elevated PRL levels either on (n = 3) or off (n = 5) dopamine agonist therapy. A meta-analysis by Yang and colleagues[45] evaluated the rates of remission in acromegaly treated with SRS and found that following SRS, the rate of cure was approximately 48% to 53%. At Stanford University, the authors have reported their initial experience of using SRS to treat acromegaly caused by growth hormone hypersecretion by a pituitary somatotroph adenoma.[46] CyberKnife SRS, delivered as a single session (n = 5), 2 sessions (n = 3), or 3 sessions (n = 1), resulted in complete biochemical remission in 4 (44.4%) patients and in biochemical control with the concomitant use of a somatostatin analogue in an additional patient.[46] Rates of complications following SRS for acromegaly, including new anterior pituitary deficits (0%–50%) and worsening of visual acuity or fields (0%–4%), were comparable with other tumor types receiving SRS.[47] SRS can be a useful adjunct to surgical treatment in Cushing disease resulting from adrenocorticotrophic hormone (ACTH)–producing adenoma because failure to achieve remission or tumor recurrence occurs in up to 30% following successful transsphenoidal resection.[48] Many reports showed ACTH normalization rates of approximately 40% to 65% following SRS.[49] Jagannathan and colleagues[50] reported on 90 patients with Cushing disease undergoing SRS with a mean dose of 23 Gy (median 25 Gy) and a mean endocrine follow-up of 45 months. They reported normalization of 24-hour urinary-free cortisol in 54% of patients, with an average time to remission of 13 months (range 2–67 months).[50] Twenty percent of their patients demonstrated tumor recurrence between 6 and 60 months after SRS, suggesting the need for extended follow-up in patients with Cushing disease to monitor for tumor recurrence.[50] Although there are ample data demonstrating the efficacy of single-session SRS for the treatment of the aforementioned functional adenomas, there remains room for the study of multi-session SRS scheduling in comparing efficacy and complication rates.

Overall, SRS is preferable to EBRT for a variety of reasons. SRS is more convenient for patients because it is performed as a single-day, outpatient-based procedure as opposed to EBRT, which is typically performed over 5 to 6 weeks. Biochemical remission seems to be shorter after SRS for patients with hormone-secreting tumors. Kong and colleagues[38] compared the efficacy of EBRT (64 patients, mean dose 50.4 Gy) and single-fraction SRS (61 patients, mean dose 25.1 Gy) in

125 patients with pituitary adenomas and showed a shorter time to biochemical remission after SRS (median time to remission 26 months vs 63 months). The potential to normalize hormone levels more rapidly makes SRS more preferable in patients with either acromegaly or Cushing disease in order to minimize the metabolic consequences of these conditions. The incidence of new pituitary deficits can be higher after EBRT compared with SRS (60%–80% vs 10%–40%).[51] SRS has a lower incidence of radiation-induced neoplasms compared with EBRT.[52,53] In fact, Rowe and colleagues,[54] from the National Center for Stereotactic Radiosurgery in Sheffield, found no difference in incidence in their radiosurgical patients compared with the age- and sex-adjusted national cohort of 5000 patients and more than 30,000 patient-years of follow-up.

COMPLICATIONS AND CONCERNS

SRS, as with all forms of radiotherapy, is associated with a range of toxicities in the management of meningiomas, including radiation necrosis, peritumoral edema, hemiparesis, cranial nerve deficits, vascular occlusion, and delayed hydrocephalus.[24,55,56] Locations of meningiomas may dictate the risk for radiation-induced complications, such is the case for convexity and parasagittal meningiomas. At Stanford University, the authors reported on 102 patients (111 tumors) with supratentorial meningiomas treated with CyberKnife stereotactic radiosurgery.[24] The authors noted that patients with parasagittal meningiomas were more than 4 times as likely to develop symptomatic edema after SRS when compared with patients with meningiomas in nonmidline supratentorial locations.[24] The 6-, 12-, and 18-month actuarial rates of symptomatic edema development were significantly greater for patients with parasagittal meningiomas than for patients with nonparasagittal meningiomas (17.8% vs 1.3%, 25.4% vs 5.8%, and 35.2% vs 7.8%, respectively).[24] These observations were consistent with those at the Mayo Clinic where complications occurred more frequently in patients with supratentorial tumors (44%) compared with patients with skull-base tumors (13%).[28] Tumor size is another risk factor for SRS complications. Although equivalent tumor control rates could be achieved for large tumors, there is an associated high rate of complications approaching 23%.[57] In the authors' experience, glucocorticoids can be used to relieve peritumoral edema after multi-session SRS. Kondziolka and colleagues[58] reported similar symptom resolution in single-session SRS in all their patients with peritumoral edema who were treated with steroids.

Multi-session radiosurgery may reduce the incidence of peritumoral edema, but no direct comparison studies have been made between single-session and multi-session SRS meningioma treatments.

In the treatment of pituitary adenoma with SRS, pituitary suppressive medications taken at the time of radiosurgery can negatively impact the chance of biochemical remission. Multiple studies have confirmed that pituitary suppressive medications adversely affect endocrine outcomes.[9,59,60] It stands to reason that even with multi-session scheduling of SRS, the same mechanism could hinder biochemical remission. Therefore, it is recommended that patients should not take pituitary suppressive medications for several months before SRS.

Radiation-induced neoplasms caused by SRS for benign intracranial neoplasms may be concerning to patients in light of such risk from conventional radiation. However, Rowe and colleagues[54] reported no increased risk of new tumor formation in the SRS-treated population versus healthy controls; the use of radiation can elicit safety concerns. No data exist that compare the risk of malignant transformation between single-session and multi-session SRS.

The theory behind multi-session SRS to limit the damage to adjacent structures, such is the case of the cochlear nerve for vestibular schwannomas, has also not been definitively proven. However, the idea of multi-session SRS is attractive because of its theoretical potential to limit facial nerve dysfunction and maximize hearing preservation. To that end, comparisons between single-session and multi-session SRS are warranted to compare efficacy and safety in treating the variety of benign intracranial tumors using standardized outcome measurements.

SUMMARY

Multi-session SRS enables a high dose per fraction to be delivered to the tumor bed with rapid dose falloff that allows for sparing of critical structures, resulting in less radiation-associated toxicity. Although comparisons between single- and multi-session SRS are still emerging, data from using multi-session SRS for treating benign intracranial tumors are encouraging. The authors' efforts in treating meningioma using multi-session SRS have identified tumor location as a key determinant of risk for radiation-induced complications. Particularly, CyberKnife SRS administered in multi-sessions may reduce facial complications and hearing loss in vestibular schwannomas. Multi-session SRS is also an attractive approach in pituitary adenomas because of its potential to minimize damage to the surrounding optic apparatus.

REFERENCES

1. Leksell L. The stereotaxic method and radiosurgery of the brain. Acta Chir Scand 1951;102(4):316–9.
2. Shrieve DC, Hazard L, Boucher K, et al. Dose fractionation in stereotactic radiotherapy for parasellar meningiomas: radiobiological considerations of efficacy and optic nerve tolerance. J Neurosurg 2004;101(Suppl 3):390–5.
3. Davidson L, Fishback D, Russin JJ, et al. Postoperative gamma knife surgery for benign meningiomas of the cranial base. Neurosurg Focus 2007;23(4):E6.
4. Tuniz F, Soltys SG, Choi CY, et al. Multisession cyberknife stereotactic radiosurgery of large, benign cranial base tumors: preliminary study. Neurosurgery 2009;65(5):898–907 [discussion: 907].
5. Hall EJ, Brenner DJ. The radiobiology of radiosurgery: rationale for different treatment regimes for AVMs and malignancies. Int J Radiat Oncol Biol Phys 1993;25(2):381–5.
6. Choi CY, Soltys SG, Gibbs IC, et al. Cyberknife stereotactic radiosurgery for treatment of atypical (WHO grade II) cranial meningiomas. Neurosurgery 2010;67(5):1180–8.
7. Kondziolka D, Mousavi SH, Kano H, et al. The newly diagnosed vestibular schwannoma: radiosurgery, resection, or observation? Neurosurg Focus 2012;33(3):E8.
8. Sheehan JP, Niranjan A, Sheehan JM, et al. Stereotactic radiosurgery for pituitary adenomas: an intermediate review of its safety, efficacy, and role in the neurosurgical treatment armamentarium. J Neurosurg 2005;102(4):678–91.
9. Pollock BE, Jacob JT, Brown PD, et al. Radiosurgery of growth hormone-producing pituitary adenomas: factors associated with biochemical remission. J Neurosurg 2007;106(5):833–8.
10. Claus EB, Bondy ML, Schildkraut JM, et al. Epidemiology of intracranial meningioma. Neurosurgery 2005;57(6):1088–95 [discussion: 1088–95].
11. Sughrue ME, Rutkowski MJ, Aranda D, et al. Treatment decision making based on the published natural history and growth rate of small meningiomas. J Neurosurg 2010;113(5):1036–42.
12. Mirimanoff RO, Dosoretz DE, Linggood RM, et al. Meningioma: analysis of recurrence and progression following neurosurgical resection. J Neurosurg 1985;62(1):18–24.
13. Stafford SL, Perry A, Suman VJ, et al. Primarily resected meningiomas: outcome and prognostic

factors in 581 Mayo Clinic patients, 1978 through 1988. Mayo Clin Proc 1998;73(10):936–42.

14. DiBiase SJ, Kwok Y, Yovino S, et al. Factors predicting local tumor control after gamma knife stereotactic radiosurgery for benign intracranial meningiomas. Int J Radiat Oncol Biol Phys 2004; 60(5):1515–9.

15. Roche PH, Pellet W, Fuentes S, et al. Gamma knife radiosurgical management of petroclival meningiomas results and indications. Acta Neurochir (Wien) 2003;145(10):883–8 [discussion: 888].

16. Kreil W, Luggin J, Fuchs I, et al. Long term experience of gamma knife radiosurgery for benign skull base meningiomas. J Neurol Neurosurg Psychiatry 2005;76(10):1425–30.

17. Iwai Y, Yamanaka K, Ikeda H. Gamma Knife radiosurgery for skull base meningioma: long-term results of low-dose treatment. J Neurosurg 2008; 109(5):804–10.

18. Pollock BE, Stafford SL, Utter A, et al. Stereotactic radiosurgery provides equivalent tumor control to Simpson Grade 1 resection for patients with small- to medium-size meningiomas. Int J Radiat Oncol Biol Phys 2003;55(4):1000–5.

19. Zachenhofer I, Wolfsberger S, Aichholzer M, et al. Gamma-knife radiosurgery for cranial base meningiomas: experience of tumor control, clinical course, and morbidity in a follow-up of more than 8 years. Neurosurgery 2006;58(1):28–36 [discussion: 28–36].

20. Starke RM, Williams BJ, Hiles C, et al. Gamma knife surgery for skull base meningiomas. J Neurosurg 2012;116(3):588–97.

21. Lee JY, Niranjan A, McInerney J, et al. Stereotactic radiosurgery providing long-term tumor control of cavernous sinus meningiomas. J Neurosurg 2002; 97(1):65–72.

22. Pollock BE, Stafford SL. Results of stereotactic radiosurgery for patients with imaging defined cavernous sinus meningiomas. Int J Radiat Oncol Biol Phys 2005;62(5):1427–31.

23. Kondziolka D, Mathieu D, Lunsford LD, et al. Radiosurgery as definitive management of intracranial meningiomas. Neurosurgery 2008;62(1):53–8 [discussion: 58–60].

24. Patil CG, Hoang S, Borchers DJ 3rd, et al. Predictors of peritumoral edema after stereotactic radiosurgery of supratentorial meningiomas. Neurosurgery 2008;63(3):435–40 [discussion: 440–2].

25. Myrseth E, Moller P, Pedersen PH, et al. Vestibular schwannomas: clinical results and quality of life after microsurgery or gamma knife radiosurgery. Neurosurgery 2005;56(5):927–35 [discussion: 927–35].

26. Pollock BE, Lunsford LD, Kondziolka D, et al. Outcome analysis of acoustic neuroma management: a comparison of microsurgery and stereotactic radiosurgery. Neurosurgery 1995;36(1):215–24 [discussion: 224–9].

27. Regis J, Pellet W, Delsanti C, et al. Functional outcome after gamma knife surgery or microsurgery for vestibular schwannomas. J Neurosurg 2002;97(5):1091–100.

28. Pollock BE. Stereotactic radiosurgery of benign intracranial tumors. J Neurooncol 2009;92(3): 337–43.

29. Kondziolka D, Lunsford LD, McLaughlin MR, et al. Long-term outcomes after radiosurgery for acoustic neuromas. N Engl J Med 1998;339(20): 1426–33.

30. Linskey ME, Lunsford LD, Flickinger JC. Radiosurgery for acoustic neurinomas: early experience. Neurosurgery 1990;26(5):736–44 [discussion: 744–5].

31. Lunsford LD, Linskey ME. Stereotactic radiosurgery in the treatment of patients with acoustic tumors. Otolaryngol Clin North Am 1992;25(2):471–91.

32. Massager N, Nissim O, Delbrouck C, et al. Irradiation of cochlear structures during vestibular schwannoma radiosurgery and associated hearing outcome. J Neurosurg 2007;107(4):733–9.

33. Thomas C, Di Maio S, Ma R, et al. Hearing preservation following fractionated stereotactic radiotherapy for vestibular schwannomas: prognostic implications of cochlear dose. J Neurosurg 2007; 107(5):917–26.

34. Chang SD, Gibbs IC, Sakamoto GT, et al. Staged stereotactic irradiation for acoustic neuroma. Neurosurgery 2005;56(6):1254–61 [discussion: 1261–3].

35. Hansasuta A, Choi CY, Gibbs IC, et al. Multisession stereotactic radiosurgery for vestibular schwannomas: single-institution experience with 383 cases. Neurosurgery 2011;69(6):1200–9.

36. Pollock BE, Driscoll CL, Foote RL, et al. Patient outcomes after vestibular schwannoma management: a prospective comparison of microsurgical resection and stereotactic radiosurgery. Neurosurgery 2006;59(1):77–85 [discussion: 77–85].

37. Chopra R, Kondziolka D, Niranjan A, et al. Long-term follow-up of acoustic schwannoma radiosurgery with marginal tumor doses of 12 to 13 Gy. Int J Radiat Oncol Biol Phys 2007;68(3): 845–51.

38. Kong DS, Lee JI, Lim do H, et al. The efficacy of fractionated radiotherapy and stereotactic radiosurgery for pituitary adenomas: long-term results of 125 consecutive patients treated in a single institution. Cancer 2007;110(4):854–60.

39. Tanaka S, Link MJ, Brown PD, et al. Gamma knife radiosurgery for patients with prolactin-secreting pituitary adenomas. World Neurosurg 2010;74(1): 147–52.

40. Gopalan R, Schlesinger D, Vance ML, et al. Long-term outcomes after Gamma Knife radiosurgery for patients with a nonfunctioning pituitary adenoma. Neurosurgery 2011;69(2):284–93.

41. Stafford SL, Pollock BE, Leavitt JA, et al. A study on the radiation tolerance of the optic nerves and chiasm after stereotactic radiosurgery. Int J Radiat Oncol Biol Phys 2003;55(5):1177–81.

42. Adler JR Jr, Gibbs IC, Puataweepong P, et al. Visual field preservation after multisession cyberknife radiosurgery for perioptic lesions. Neurosurgery 2006;59(2):244–54 [discussion: 244–54].

43. Pollock BE, Cochran J, Natt N, et al. Gamma knife radiosurgery for patients with nonfunctioning pituitary adenomas: results from a 15-year experience. Int J Radiat Oncol Biol Phys 2008;70(5): 1325–9.

44. Starke RM, Williams BJ, Jane JA Jr, et al. Gamma Knife surgery for patients with nonfunctioning pituitary macroadenomas: predictors of tumor control, neurological deficits, and hypopituitarism. J Neurosurg 2012;117(1):129–35.

45. Yang I, Kim W, De Salles A, et al. A systematic analysis of disease control in acromegaly treated with radiosurgery. Neurosurg Focus 2010;29(4):E13.

46. Roberts BK, Ouyang DL, Lad SP, et al. Efficacy and safety of CyberKnife radiosurgery for acromegaly. Pituitary 2007;10(1):19–25.

47. Ronchi CL, Attanasio R, Verrua E, et al. Efficacy and tolerability of gamma knife radiosurgery in acromegaly: a 10-year follow-up study. Clin Endocrinol (Oxf) 2009;71(6):846–52.

48. Patil CG, Prevedello DM, Lad SP, et al. Late recurrences of Cushing's disease after initial successful transsphenoidal surgery. J Clin Endocrinol Metab 2008;93(2):358–62.

49. Kim W, Clelland C, Yang I, et al. Comprehensive review of stereotactic radiosurgery for medically and surgically refractory pituitary adenomas. Surg Neurol Int 2012;3(Suppl 2):S79–89.

50. Jagannathan J, Sheehan JP, Pouratian N, et al. Gamma Knife surgery for Cushing's disease. J Neurosurg 2007;106(6):980–7.

51. Pollock BE. Comparing radiation therapy and radiosurgery for pituitary adenoma patients. World Neurosurg 2012;78(1–2):58–9.

52. Breen P, Flickinger JC, Kondziolka D, et al. Radiotherapy for nonfunctional pituitary adenoma: analysis of long-term tumor control. J Neurosurg 1998;89(6):933–8.

53. Minniti G, Traish D, Ashley S, et al. Risk of second brain tumor after conservative surgery and radiotherapy for pituitary adenoma: update after an additional 10 years. J Clin Endocrinol Metab 2005;90(2):800–4.

54. Rowe J, Grainger A, Walton L, et al. Risk of malignancy after gamma knife stereotactic radiosurgery. Neurosurgery 2007;60(1):60–5 [discussion: 65–6].

55. Barami K, Grow A, Brem S, et al. Vascular complications after radiosurgery for meningiomas. Neurosurg Focus 2007;22(3):E9.

56. Girvigian MR, Chen JC, Rahimian J, et al. Comparison of early complications for patients with convexity and parasagittal meningiomas treated with either stereotactic radiosurgery or fractionated stereotactic radiotherapy. Neurosurgery 2008; 62(Suppl 5):A19–27 [discussion: A27–8].

57. Bledsoe JM, Link MJ, Stafford SL, et al. Radiosurgery for large-volume (>10 cm3) benign meningiomas. J Neurosurg 2010;112(5):951–6.

58. Kondziolka D, Flickinger JC, Perez B. Judicious resection and/or radiosurgery for parasagittal meningiomas: outcomes from a multicenter review. Gamma Knife Meningioma Study Group. Neurosurgery 1998;43(3):405–13 [discussion: 413–4].

59. Jagannathan J, Sheehan JP, Pouratian N, et al. Gamma knife radiosurgery for acromegaly: outcomes after failed transsphenoidal surgery. Neurosurgery 2008;62(6):1262–9 [discussion: 1269–70].

60. Pouratian N, Sheehan J, Jagannathan J, et al. Gamma knife radiosurgery for medically and surgically refractory prolactinomas. Neurosurgery 2006; 59(2):255–66 [discussion: 255–66].

Stereotactic Radiosurgery of Intracranial Chordomas, Chondrosarcomas, and Glomus Tumors

Hideyuki Kano, MD, PhD*, L. Dade Lunsford, MD

KEYWORDS

- Chordoma • Chondrosarcoma • Glomus tumor • Skull base • Stereotactic radiosurgery
- Gamma knife

KEY POINTS

- Chordomas and chondrosarcomas are rare, slow-glowing, locally aggressive tumors with high recurrence rates that may prove disabling or fatal.
- Patients with intracranial chordomas and chondrosarcomas often require multimodality treatment, including surgical resection, fractionated radiation therapy, and stereotactic radiosurgery (SRS).
- SRS is an important management option for patients with recurrent or residual chordomas and chondrosarcomas that failed to respond to initial surgical resection and adjuvant radiation therapy.
- The local tumor control rate and prognosis is generally better for patients with chondrosarcomas than for those with chordomas.
- SRS can be used as an up-front treatment or as an adjuvant treatment for patients with recurrent or residual glomus jugulare tumors after surgical resection.

INTRODUCTION

Chordomas are slowly-growing, locally aggressive tumors that arise from embryonic remnants of the notochord and show a dural epithelial-mesenchymal differentiation.[1] They arise from the sacrococcygeal region in 50% to 60% of patients, from the skull base region in 25% to 35%, and from the vertebrae in 15%.[2] The natural history of untreated clival chordomas is dismal, with a mean survival of less than 1 year.[3] Neurologic deficits tend to vary based on the location of the tumor. An abducens nerve deficit causing diplopia is the most frequent presenting sign.[4,5]

CHORDOMAS
Therapeutic Options

Aggressive initial management, beginning with radical resection when possible and followed by fractionated radiation therapy or radiosurgery, improves overall outcome.[6] Earlier recognition of these tumors[7–10] facilitates aggressive therapy. Complete resection without significant morbidity is rarely feasible because these tumors tend to encase critical vessels and cranial nerves, or adhere to the brainstem.[11–15] The recurrence rate, even after virtually complete resection, remains high.[16,17] Recurrent tumors are even more challenging for

Disclosures: Dr Lunsford is a consultant for and a stockholder of AB Elekta.
Department of Neurological Surgery, The Center for Image-Guided Neurosurgery, UPMC Presbyterian, University of Pittsburgh School of Medicine, University of Pittsburgh, Suite B-400, 200 Lothrop Street, Pittsburgh, PA 15213, USA
* Corresponding author.
E-mail address: kanoh@upmc.edu

Neurosurg Clin N Am 24 (2013) 553–560
http://dx.doi.org/10.1016/j.nec.2013.05.009
1042-3680/13/$ – see front matter © 2013 Elsevier Inc. All rights reserved.

extirpation. Most patients undergo adjuvant radiation therapy to reduce the risk of tumor recurrence. Chordomas are considered radioresistant tumors that require total fractionated radiation therapy doses in excess of 60 Gy to reduce recurrence rates.[1] Fractionated stereotactic radiation therapy using high-energy photons or fractionated charged particle radiation (most often protons) are the 2 most commonly administered forms of radiation for chordomas.[18–22] Prior reports comparing results of photon irradiation with proton beam therapy rarely take into account the more recent evolution of photon-based treatments in which energies are higher, and targeting and delivery methods have been enhanced. Regardless of the radiation modality, the maximum dose of radiation that can be safely delivered is limited by the tolerance of the surrounding critical cranial nerve, brainstem, or temporal lobe structures.[23–26]

Based on the principle of Bragg peak deposition of energy that reduces exit dose, fractionated, charged-particle radiation delivered by protons or carbon ions is thought by some to deliver a more radiobiologically potent dose to the tumor. The Bragg peak effect results in a rapid energy deposition at the target volume, with a steep dose drop-off beyond the target volume treated.[27] With proton beam radiation therapy, doses greater than 70 cobalt gray equivalent (CGE) are prescribed. CGE is an empiric measure of estimated radiation effect obtained through multiplying the conventional photon radiation dose in Gy by 1.2, a value that has been postulated but unproven to be the potential radiobiological advantage of proton Bragg peak radiation therapy. Published data indicate that experienced centers may achieve local tumor control rates of 67% to 88% at 3 years, 46% to 73% at 5 years, and 54% at 10 years. The overall survival rates are 67% to 81% at 5 years and 54% at 10 years.[28] These results are often interpreted as superior to those reported for chordomas treated by older fractionated photon radiation therapy techniques before the era of intensity-modulated radiation therapy (IMRT).[27] Using carbon ion therapy, Castro and colleagues[29] treated 53 patients with doses of 60 to 80 CGE. They reported 5-year local tumor control and overall survival rates of 63% and 75%, respectively. Schulz-Ertner and colleagues[30] reported that 96 patients with chordoma who underwent carbon ion fractionated radiation therapy showed 5-year local tumor control and overall survival rates of 70% and 88.5%, respectively. Late toxicity consisted of optic nerve neuropathy Radiation Therapy Oncology Group (RTOG)/European Organisation for Research and Treatment of Cancer (EORTC) grade 3 in 4.1% of the patients. Minor temporal lobe injury (RTOG/ EORTC grade 1–2) occurred in 7.2% of the patients.

Noel and colleagues[31] reported the results of combined fractionated photon and proton radiation therapy in 90 patients with either chordomas ($n = 64$) or chondrosarcomas ($n = 26$) of the skull base. The tumors were treated to a median total dose of 67 CGE (range, 22–70 CGE). Photons represented two-thirds of the total delivered dose, and protons represented one-third. At a median follow-up of 34 months, local tumor control was achieved in 65 patients (72%). All 90 patients developed immediate adverse radiation effects, usually mild. However, 6% reported late grade III or IV radiation toxicities, including cranial nerve deficits and visual loss. Proton fractionated radiation therapy remains a relatively expensive strategy that is available in a limited but increasing number of facilities in the United States and abroad.

Clinical Outcomes of Stereotactic Radiosurgery

Stereotactic radiosurgery (SRS) is a surgical technique designed to achieve a greater radiobiological effect than conventional 3-dimensional conformal radiation therapy or IMRT. SRS has been used as a minimally invasive primary or adjuvant management option for chordomas (**Fig. 1**, **Table 1**).[32–34] SRS using the Leksell Gamma Knife (Elekta Inc, Norcross, GA) is a surgical procedure that delivers cross-fired photon radiation generated from the decay of cobalt 60 sources in a single wheels-in-to-wheels-out procedure. Using linear accelerator technologies, such as the Accuray CyberKnife (Accuray, Sunnyvale, CA), SRS may be delivered in up to 5 treatment sessions. Delivery of such highly focused radiation in 1 to 5 sessions significantly increases the radiobiological effect of SRS compared with conventional fractionated radiation therapy. Using methods to evaluate radiobiological effects, the center of the tumor may receive a radiobiological effect 4 times of what can be safely delivered using conventional fractionated radiation or IMRT. SRS seems especially valuable for the treatment of relatively small residual or recurrent chordomas after prior surgical resection. SRS has been frequently added as a radiobiological boost to conventional fractionated radiation therapy. Krishnan and colleagues[33] treated 25 patients with cranial base chordoma with SRS using a median tumor margin dose of 15 Gy. The 5-year treated tumor control rate was 52% at a median follow-up of 4.5 years. Hasegawa and colleagues[32] performed SRS on 27 patients with chordoma with median tumor

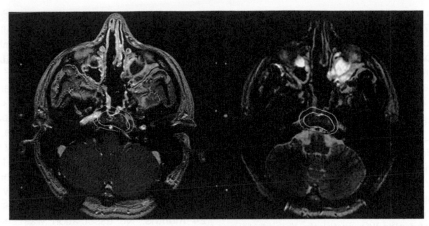

Fig. 1. T1-weighted contrast-enhanced (*left*) and T2-weighted (*right*) axial magnetic resonance imaging scan of residual chordoma involving clivus, showing the stereotactic radiosurgery target with a margin dose of 18 Gy.

margin doses of 14 Gy. They noted 5-year local tumor control and overall survival rates of 42% and 80%, respectively, at a median follow-up of 59 months. In their series, only tumor volumes of less than 20 cm³ were significantly associated with a longer progression-free survival (PFS). Liu and colleagues[35] reported on 28 patients with residual skull base chordoma who underwent SRS with median margin dose of 12.7 Gy. The average follow-up was 28 months and the mean tumor volume was 11.4 ± 7.4 cm³. The 5-year overall survival and in-field tumor control rates were 75.8% and 21.4%, respectively. No serious adverse radiation effects (AREs) were reported.

Kano and colleagues[36] reported that 6 participating centers of the North American Gamma Knife Consortium identified 71 patients who underwent Gamma Knife SRS for chordomas. The median patient age was 45 years (range, 7–80 years). The median SRS target volume was 7.1 cm³ (range, 0.9–109.0 cm³) and the median tumor margin dose was 15.0 Gy (range, 9–25 Gy). At a median

follow-up of 5 years after SRS (range, 0.6–14.0 years), 23 patients died because of tumor progression. The 5-year actuarial overall survival after SRS for the entire group was 80%. Tumor control was higher (93%) in patients who had not undergone prior fractionated radiation therapy ($n = 50$). Tumor control was reduced to 43% in patients who underwent prior fractionated radiation therapy ($n = 21$). Factors associated with longer patient survival included younger age, longer interval between initial diagnosis and SRS, no prior radiation therapy, fewer than 2 cranial nerve deficits, and smaller total tumor volumes. The 5-year treated tumor control rates after SRS for the entire group was 66% (69% for the no prior fractionated radiation therapy group and 62% for the prior fractionated radiation therapy group). Significant factors associated with reduced tumor control included older age, recurrent tumors, prior fractionated radiation therapy, and larger tumor volumes. Of 57 patients with pretreatment neurologic deficits, 17 (30%) experienced neurologic improvement. Of 65

Table 1
Studies and patient characteristics in published series of chordoma treated with SRS

Reference	N	Radiation	Median Margin Dose (range)	Tumor Volume	% Local Control	% Survival	Median Follow-up (mo)
Krishnan et al,[33] 2005	19	SRS ± RT	15.0 Gy (10.0–20.0 Gy) ± 50.4 Gy (45.0–54.0 Gy)	14.4 cm³	4 y: 55	NA	58
Hasegawa et al,[32] 2007	27	SRS	14 Gy (9–20 Gy)	19.7 cm³	5 y: 72 10 y: 72	5 y: 84 10 y: 67	59
Liu et al,[35] 2008	31	SRS	12.7 Gy (10.0–16.0 Gy)	11.4 cm³	3 y: 64 5 y: 21	3 y: 91 5 y: 76	28
Kano et al,[36] 2011	71	SRS ± RT	15 Gy (9–25 Gy)	7.1 cm³	3 y: 79 5 y: 66	5 y: 80 7 y: 69	60

Abbreviations: NA, not available; RT, fractionated radiation therapy.

patients with clinical follow-up, 31 (48%) remained stable, but 17 (26%) eventually had deterioration in neurologic function. Deterioration was related to treated tumor progression in 8 patients, adjacent tumor progression in 3, treatment-associated AREs in 4, and both treated tumor progression and AREs in 2.

Summary

Maximal safe resection should be the primary initial treatment for chordomas. After recovery from surgery, fractionated Bragg peak proton radiation therapy at an experienced center remains an option for the additional treatment of chordomas. Careful planning and reduction of dose delivered to adjacent critical structures are critical components, whether using particle beam or modern fractionated photon radiation techniques. Long-term evaluation of neurocognitive effects are warranted because of the relatively higher dose that may be delivered via the entrance pathway within the temporal lobes. SRS after surgical resection also provides a reasonable benefit-to-risk profile for small- to medium-sized chordomas. SRS is an important option for patients with recurrent tumors that failed to respond to initial surgical resection. Current data suggest that it might well supplant radiation therapy as the next best option for residual smaller-volume tumors.

CHONDROSARCOMA

Chondrosarcomas are relatively slow-growing, locally invasive tumors that usually do not metastasize until very late in the natural history.[12] Cranial chondrosarcomas originate from primitive mesenchymal cells within the cartilaginous matrix of the skull base.[2] The imaging features and clinical presentations of patients harboring either chordomas or chondrosarcomas are similar. Chordomas have a tendency to cause brainstem compression because they arise from the clivus, whereas chondrosarcomas tend to affect the lower cranial nerves because they frequently originate from the occipitotemporal bone synchondrosis.[37] The most common presenting symptom of chondrosarcoma is diplopia, secondary to an abducens nerve palsy.[38] Using imaging alone to distinguish chondrosarcomas from chordomas is often difficult but important, because the prognosis is generally considered better for chondrosarcomas.[28,39]

Therapeutic Options

Chondrosarcomas are rarely completely resectable, and additional management options must be considered for residual tumors.[40,41] Gay and colleagues[12] reported a 90% overall survival at 5 years for 14 patients who underwent either skull base surgery or surgery followed by radiation therapy. Crockard and colleagues[42] reported a 93% 5-year survival rate for 17 patients who underwent surgery alone. Bloch and colleagues[43] found a recurrence rate of 44% in patients who underwent surgical resection alone, compared with 9% in patients who had surgery followed by radiation therapy. A recent review of the literature described 560 patients with intracranial chondrosarcomas, which were associated with a 5-year mortality rate of 11.5% and a median survival of 24 months. No association was seen between the rate of recurrence and the histologic grade of the tumor.[43] In a study of 8 patients with chondrosarcomas and 8 with chordomas of the skull base who underwent proton radiation therapy, Fuji and colleagues[44] reported a local control rate at 3 years of 86% and a median follow-up of 42 months. Other studies using proton radiation therapy have also reported overall survival and local tumor control rates at 5 years to be greater than 90%.[45–47]

Clinical Outcomes of SRS

Relatively few data exist to define the use of SRS in the multimodal management of chondrosarcoma (Fig. 2, Table 2). SRS has been shown to result in less toxicity to surrounding structures and have fewer complications than fractionated radiation therapy in the management of chondrosarcomas. Koga and colleagues[48] reported the results of 4 patients who had surgical resection followed by SRS at a median follow-up of 99 months. Three of the patients, who received margin doses of 15, 16, and 20 Gy, had no change in tumor size during follow-up. One patient who received a lower tumor margin dose of 12 Gy developed tumor recurrence 100 months after SRS. Hasegawa and colleagues[32] studied 30 patients with chordomas and 7 patients with chondrosarcomas who underwent SRS. The 5-year PFS rate in patients with low-grade chondrosarcomas was 76%. A tumor volume of less than 20 mL significantly improved PFS. Krishnan and colleagues[33] reported that 4 patients with chondrosarcomas who underwent SRS had tumor control at 5 years.

Iyer and colleagues[49] studied 22 patients who underwent Gamma Knife SRS for residual or recurrent intracranial chondrosarcomas. Overall patient survival rates after SRS were 95%, 70%, and 56% at 1, 5, and 10 years, respectively. Factors associated with longer survival after SRS included a shorter interval (<6 months) between

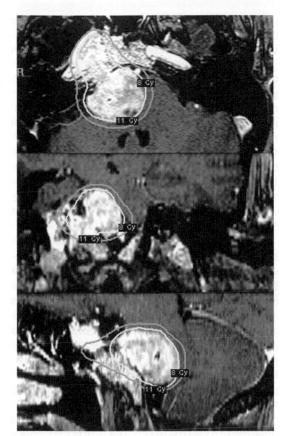

Fig. 2. T1-weighted contrast-enhanced axial (*upper*), coronal (*middle*), and sagittal (*lower*) magnetic resonance imaging scan of residual chondrosarcoma involving the right petroclival and cerebellopontine angle, showing the stereotactic radiosurgery target with a margin dose of 11 Gy.

diagnosis and SRS, age older than 40 years, and either a single or no prior resection. Treated tumor control rates were 91% at 1 year, 72% at 5 years, and 54% at 10 years. Factors associated with

longer PFS after SRS included patient age older than 40 years and no prior radiation therapy.

Summary

The ability to achieve tumor growth control of chondrosarcomas is likely to be enhanced by earlier recognition and the application of multimodal treatment in appropriate patients. Maximal safe resection should be the primary initial management of chondrosarcomas. Gamma Knife radiosurgery is a reasonable therapeutic option as an adjuvant treatment after resection in selected patients with chondrosarcomas.

GLOMUS JUGULARE TUMORS

Glomus jugulare tumors are rare, highly vascularized tumors that arise from the paraganglionic structures of the glossopharyngeal and vagal nerves. Because of their highly vascular nature and generally inaccessible anatomic location, surgical resection is often challenging. The ideal treatment for patients with a glomus tumor remains controversial. Treatment options include surgical resection, endovascular embolization, fractionated radiation therapy, and SRS alone or in combination.

Clinical Outcomes of SRS

Liscak and colleagues[50] reported on 52 patients with glomus jugulare tumors treated with SRS (**Fig. 3**, **Table 3**); 24 had prior surgical resection, 14 had prior embolization, and 5 had prior RT. The median tumor volume was 5.7 cm³ (range, 0.5–27.0 cm³) and median margin dose was 16.5 Gy (range, 10–30 Gy). All patients had tumor control at a median of 24 months. The neurologic symptom control rate was 96%. Ivan and

Table 2
Studies and patient characteristics in published series of chondrosarcoma treated with SRS

Reference	N	Radiation	Median Margin Dose	Tumor Volume	% Local Control	% Survival	Median Follow-up (mo)
Krishnan et al,[33] 2005	4	SRS	15 Gy	14.4 cm³	5 y: 100	NA	58
Hasegawa et al,[32] 2007	7	SRS	14 Gy	19.7 cm³	5 y: 76 10 y: 67	5 y: 90 10 y: 53	59
Cho et al,[54] 2008	11	SRS ± RT	12.7 Gy ± 58.2 Gy	3.7 cm³	5 y: 89 10 y: 80	5 y: 100 10 y: 100	56
Koga et al,[48] 2010	4	SRS	15.6 Gy	NA	5 y: 100	NA	65
Iyer et al,[49] 2012	22	SRS ± RT	15 Gy	8.0 cm³	5 y: 72 10 y: 54	5 y: 70 10 y: 56	60

Abbreviations: NA, not available; RT, fractionated radiation therapy.

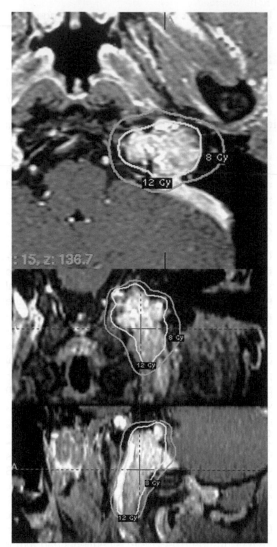

Fig. 3. T1-weighted contrast-enhanced axial (*upper*), coronal (*middle*), and sagittal (*lower*) magnetic resonance imaging scan of glomus jugulare tumor, showing the stereotactic radiosurgery target with a margin dose of 12 Gy.

colleagues[51] reported a meta-analysis of tumor control and morbidity for patients with glomus jugulare tumors. They identified 869 patients with glomus jugulare tumors from 46 publications. Patients underwent gross total resection alone had a tumor control rate of 86% at a mean follow-up of 88 months. Patients who underwent subtotal resection followed by SRS had a tumor control rate of 71% at a mean follow-up of 96 months. Patients who underwent SRS alone had a tumor control rate of 95% at a mean follow-up of 71 months. Patients who underwent gross total resection sustained worse rates of cranial nerve (CN) deficits with regard to CN IX–XI than those who underwent SRS alone.

In a meta-analysis of 19 studies involving 335 patients with glomus jugulare tumors who underwent SRS, Guss and colleagues[52] reported that 97% of patients experienced tumor control and 95% experienced clinical control. Sheehan and colleagues[53] performed a large retrospective multicenter study of Gamma Knife SRS for glomus jugular tumors, involving 134 procedures in 132 patients, with a median follow-up of 50.5 months. Prior resection was performed in 51 patients, and prior fractionated radiation therapy was performed in 6 patients. The median tumor volume was 5.5 cm^3 (range, 0.6–58.6 cm^3). The median margin dose was 15 Gy (10–18 Gy). The 5-year tumor control rate was 88% after SRS. Absence of trigeminal nerve dysfunction at the time of radiosurgery and higher number of isocenters were significantly associated with PFS. Patients showing new or progressive cranial nerve deficits were also likely to show tumor progression. Pulsatile tinnitus improved in 49% of patients who reported it at presentation. New or progressive cranial nerve deficits were noted in 15% of patients, and improvement in preexisting cranial nerve deficits was observed in 11% of patients. No patient died as a result of tumor progression.

Table 3
Studies and patient characteristics in published series of glomus jugulare tumor treated with SRS

Reference	N	Radiation	Median Margin Dose	Tumor Volume	% Local Control	% Symptom Control	Median Follow-up (mo)
Liscak et al,[50] 1999	66	SRS ± RT	16.5 Gy	5.7 cm^3	100	96	24
Pollock et al,[55] 2004	42	SRS	14.9 Gy	19.7 cm^3	97	NA	44
Gerosa et al,[56] 2006	20	SRS	17.5 Gy	7 cm^3	100	90	50
Genc et al,[57] 2010	18	SRS	15.6 Gy	5.5 cm^3	94	94	53
Sheehan et al,[53] 2012	134	SRS ± RT	15 Gy	5.5 cm^3	92.7	85	50.5

Abbreviations: NA, not available; RT, fractionated radiation therapy.

Summary

SRS affords a high rate of local tumor control and a low risk of neurologic complications for patients with glomus jugulare tumors. SRS can be used as an up-front treatment or as an additional treatment for those with recurrent or residual tumor after surgical resection.

REFERENCES

1. Chugh R, Tawbi H, Lucas DR, et al. Chordoma: the nonsarcoma primary bone tumor. Oncologist 2007; 12(11):1344–50.

2. Heffelfinger MJ, Dahlin DC, MacCarty CS, et al. Chordomas and cartilaginous tumors at the skull base. Cancer 1973;32(2):410–20.

3. Eriksson B, Gunterberg B, Kindblom LG. Chordoma. A clinicopathologic and prognostic study of a Swedish national series. Acta Orthop Scand 1981;52(1):49–58.

4. Nishigaya K, Kaneko M, Ohashi Y, et al. Intradural retroclival chordoma without bone involvement: no tumor regrowth 5 years after operation. Case report. J Neurosurg 1998;88(4):764–8.

5. Weber AL, Liebsch NJ, Sanchez R, et al. Chordomas of the skull base. Radiologic and clinical evaluation. Neuroimaging Clin N Am 1994;4(3):515–27.

6. Carpentier A, Polivka M, Blanquet A, et al. Suboccipital and cervical chordomas: the value of aggressive treatment at first presentation of the disease. J Neurosurg 2002;97(5):1070–7.

7. Anegawa T, Rai M, Hara K, et al. An unusual cervical chordoma: CT and MRI. Neuroradiology 1996; 38(5):466–7.

8. Ducou le Pointe H, Brugieres P, Chevalier X, et al. Imaging of chordomas of the mobile spine. J Neuroradiol 1991;18(3):267–76.

9. Murphy JM, Wallis F, Toland J, et al. CT and MRI appearances of a thoracic chordoma. Eur Radiol 1998;8(9):1677–9.

10. Smolders D, Wang X, Drevelengas A, et al. Value of MRI in the diagnosis of non-clival, non-sacral chordoma. Skeletal Radiol 2003;32(6):343–50.

11. al-Mefty O, Borba LA. Skull base chordomas: a management challenge. J Neurosurg 1997;86(2):182–9.

12. Gay E, Sekhar LN, Rubinstein E, et al. Chordomas and chondrosarcomas of the cranial base: results and follow-up of 60 patients. Neurosurgery 1995; 36(5):887–96 [discussion: 896–7].

13. Maira G, Pallini R, Anile C, et al. Surgical treatment of clival chordomas: the transsphenoidal approach revisited. J Neurosurg 1996;85(5):784–92.

14. Sen CN, Sekhar LN, Schramm VL, et al. Chordoma and chondrosarcoma of the cranial base: an 8-year experience. Neurosurgery 1989;25(6): 931–40 [discussion: 940–1].

15. Uttley D, Moore A, Archer DJ. Surgical management of midline skull-base tumors: a new approach. J Neurosurg 1989;71(5 Pt 1):705–10.

16. Menezes AH, Gantz BJ, Traynelis VC, et al. Cranial base chordomas. Clin Neurosurg 1997;44: 491–509.

17. Tzortzidis F, Elahi F, Wright D, et al. Patient outcome at long-term follow-up after aggressive microsurgical resection of cranial base chordomas. Neurosurgery 2006;59(2):230–7 [discussion: 230–7].

18. Igaki H, Tokuuye K, Okumura T, et al. Clinical results of proton beam therapy for skull base chordoma. Int J Radiat Oncol Biol Phys 2004;60(4): 1120–6.

19. Noel G, Feuvret L, Calugaru V, et al. Chordomas of the base of the skull and upper cervical spine. One hundred patients irradiated by a 3D conformal technique combining photon and proton beams. Acta Oncol 2005;44(7):700–8.

20. Schulz-Ertner D, Nikoghosyan A, Thilmann C, et al. Results of carbon ion radiotherapy in 152 patients. Int J Radiat Oncol Biol Phys 2004;58(2):631–40.

21. Terahara A, Niemierko A, Goitein M, et al. Analysis of the relationship between tumor dose inhomogeneity and local control in patients with skull base chordoma. Int J Radiat Oncol Biol Phys 1999; 45(2):351–8.

22. Weber DC, Rutz HP, Pedroni ES, et al. Results of spot-scanning proton radiation therapy for chordoma and chondrosarcoma of the skull base: the Paul Scherrer Institut experience. Int J Radiat Oncol Biol Phys 2005;63(2):401–9.

23. Debus J, Hug EB, Liebsch NJ, et al. Brainstem tolerance to conformal radiotherapy of skull base tumors. Int J Radiat Oncol Biol Phys 1997;39(5): 967–75.

24. Habrand IL, Austin-Seymour M, Birnbaum S, et al. Neurovisual outcome following proton radiation therapy. Int J Radiat Oncol Biol Phys 1989;16(6): 1601–6.

25. Pai HH, Thornton A, Katznelson L, et al. Hypothalamic/pituitary function following high-dose conformal radiotherapy to the base of skull: demonstration of a dose-effect relationship using dose-volume histogram analysis. Int J Radiat Oncol Biol Phys 2001;49(4):1079–92.

26. Slater JD, Austin-Seymour M, Munzenrider J, et al. Endocrine function following high dose proton therapy for tumors of the upper clivus. Int J Radiat Oncol Biol Phys 1988;15(3):607–11.

27. Amichetti M, Cianchetti M, Amelio D, et al. Proton therapy in chordoma of the base of the skull: a systematic review. Neurosurg Rev 2009;32(4): 403–16.

28. Munzenrider JE, Liebsch NJ. Proton therapy for tumors of the skull base. Strahlenther Onkol 1999; 175(Suppl 2):57–63.

29. Castro JR, Linstadt DE, Bahary JP, et al. Experience in charged particle irradiation of tumors of the skull base: 1977-1992. Int J Radiat Oncol Biol Phys 1994;29(4):647-55.

30. Schulz-Ertner D, Karger CP, Feuerhake A, et al. Effectiveness of carbon ion radiotherapy in the treatment of skull-base chordomas. Int J Radiat Oncol Biol Phys 2007;68(2):449-57.

31. Noel G, Feuvret L, Ferrand R, et al. Radiotherapeutic factors in the management of cervical-basal chordomas and chondrosarcomas. Neurosurgery 2004;55(6):1252-60 [discussion: 1260-2].

32. Hasegawa T, Ishii D, Kida Y, et al. Gamma knife surgery for skull base chordomas and chondrosarcomas. J Neurosurg 2007;107(4):752-7.

33. Krishnan S, Foote RL, Brown PD, et al. Radiosurgery for cranial base chordomas and chondrosarcomas. Neurosurgery 2005;56(4):777-84 [discussion: 777-84].

34. Martin JJ, Niranjan A, Kondziolka D, et al. Radiosurgery for chordomas and chondrosarcomas of the skull base. J Neurosurg 2007;107(4):758-64.

35. Liu AL, Wang ZC, Sun SB, et al. Gamma knife radiosurgery for residual skull base chordomas. Neurol Res 2008;30(6):557-61.

36. Kano H, Iqbal FO, Sheehan J, et al. Stereotactic radiosurgery for chordoma: a report from the North American gamma knife consortium. Neurosurgery 2011;68(2):379-89.

37. Volpe NJ, Liebsch NJ, Munzenrider JE, et al. Neuro-ophthalmologic findings in chordoma and chondrosarcoma of the skull base. Am J Ophthalmol 1993;115(1):97-104.

38. Bloch OG, Jian BJ, Yang I, et al. Cranial chondrosarcoma and recurrence. Skull Base 2010;20(3):149-56.

39. Goel A. Chordoma and chondrosarcoma: relationship to the internal carotid artery. Acta Neurochir (Wien) 1995;133(1-2):30-5.

40. Sekhar LN, Pranatartiharan R, Chanda A, et al. Chordomas and chondrosarcomas of the skull base: results and complications of surgical management. Neurosurg Focus 2001;10(3):E2.

41. Sen CN, Sekhar LN. The subtemporal and preauricular infratemporal approach to intradural structures ventral to the brain stem. J Neurosurg 1990;73(3):345-54.

42. Crockard HA, Cheeseman A, Steel T, et al. A multidisciplinary team approach to skull base chondrosarcomas. J Neurosurg 2001;95(2):184-9.

43. Bloch OG, Jian BJ, Yang I, et al. A systematic review of intracranial chondrosarcoma and survival. J Clin Neurosci 2009;16(12):1547-51.

44. Fuji H, Nakasu Y, Ishida Y, et al. Feasibility of proton beam therapy for chordoma and chondrosarcoma of the skull base. Skull Base 2011;21(3):201-6.

45. Hug EB, Loredo LN, Slater JD, et al. Proton radiation therapy for chordomas and chondrosarcomas of the skull base. J Neurosurg 1999;91(3):432-9.

46. Korten AG, ter Berg HJ, Spincemaille GH, et al. Intracranial chondrosarcoma: review of the literature and report of 15 cases. J Neurol Neurosurg Psychiatry 1998;65(1):88-92.

47. Rosenberg AE, Nielsen GP, Keel SB, et al. Chondrosarcoma of the base of the skull: a clinicopathologic study of 200 cases with emphasis on its distinction from chordoma. Am J Surg Pathol 1999;23(11):1370-8.

48. Koga T, Shin M, Saito N. Treatment with high marginal dose is mandatory to achieve long-term control of skull base chordomas and chondrosarcomas by means of stereotactic radiosurgery. J Neurooncol 2010;98(2):233-8.

49. Iyer A, Kano H, Kondziolka D, et al. Stereotactic radiosurgery for intracranial chondrosarcoma. J Neurooncol 2012;108(3):535-42.

50. Liscak R, Vladyka V, Wowra B, et al. Gamma Knife radiosurgery of the glomus jugulare tumour—early multicentre experience. Acta Neurochir (Wien) 1999;141(11):1141-6.

51. Ivan ME, Sughrue ME, Clark AJ, et al. A meta-analysis of tumor control rates and treatment-related morbidity for patients with glomus jugulare tumors. J Neurosurg 2011;114(5):1299-305.

52. Guss ZD, Batra S, Limb CJ, et al. Radiosurgery of glomus jugulare tumors: a meta-analysis. Int J Radiat Oncol Biol Phys 2011;81(4):e497-502.

53. Sheehan JP, Tanaka S, Link MJ, et al. Gamma knife surgery for the management of glomus tumors: a multicenter study. J Neurosurg 2012;117(2):246-54.

54. Cho YH, Kim JH, Khang SK, et al. Chordomas and chondrosarcomas of the skull base: comparative analysis of clinical results in 30 patients. Neurosurg Rev 2008;31(1):35-43 [discussion].

55. Pollock BE. Stereotactic radiosurgery in patients with glomus jugulare tumors. Neurosurg Focus 2004;17(2):E10.

56. Gerosa M, Visca A, Rizzo P, et al. Glomus jugulare tumors: the option of gamma knife radiosurgery. Neurosurgery 2006;59(3):561-9 [discussion].

57. Genc A, Bicer A, Abacioglu U, et al. Gamma knife radiosurgery for the treatment of glomus jugulare tumors. J Neurooncol Mar 2010;97(1):101-8.

Stereotactic Radiosurgery of Intracranial Arteriovenous Malformations

William A. Friedman, MD

KEYWORDS

- Radiosurgery • Arteriovenous malformation • Linear accelerator • Gamma knife

KEY POINTS

- Surgery is the treatment of choice for arteriovenous malformations (AVMs), because only surgery can immediately eliminate the risk of hemorrhage. In those lesions that are high risk for surgery, radiosurgery is an attractive alternative, with high success rates and low complication rates.
- When one radiosurgery treatment fails, retreatment frequently produces a cure.
- The risk of bleeding after radiosurgery seems to decrease within the natural history risk range until AVM thrombosis occurs.
- The risk of permanent radiation-induced side effects after AVM radiosurgery is approximately 2%.

INTRODUCTION

Stereotactic radiosurgery is the term coined by Lars Leksell[1] to describe the application of a single, high dose of radiation to a stereotactically defined target volume. In the 1970s, reports began to appear documenting the successful obliteration of arteriovenous malformations (AVMs) with radiosurgery. When an AVM is treated with radiosurgery, a pathologic process seems to be induced that is similar to the response-to-injury model of atherosclerosis. Radiation injury to the vascular endothelium is thought to induce the proliferation of smooth muscle cells and the elaboration of extracellular collagen, which leads to progressive stenosis and obliteration of the AVM nidus, thereby eliminating the risk of hemorrhage.[2–5]

The advantages of radiosurgery, compared with microsurgical and endovascular treatments, are that it is noninvasive, has minimal risk of acute complications, and is performed as an outpatient procedure requiring no recovery time for the patient. The primary disadvantage of radiosurgery is that cure is not immediate. Although thrombosis of the lesion is achieved in most cases, it commonly does not occur until 2 or 3 years after treatment. During the interval between radiosurgical treatment and AVM thrombosis, the risk of hemorrhage remains. Another potential disadvantage of radiosurgery is possible long-term adverse effects of radiation. In addition, radiosurgery has been shown to be less effective for lesions of more than 10 cm^3 in volume. For these reasons, selection of the optimal treatment of an AVM is a complex decision requiring the input of experts in endovascular, open surgical, and radiosurgical treatment.

This article reviews the literature on radiosurgery for AVMs. Topics reviewed include radiosurgery results (gamma knife radiosurgery, particle beam radiosurgery, linear accelerator radiosurgery), hemorrhage after radiosurgery, radiation-induced complications, and repeat radiosurgery.

REPORTED EFFICACY OF AVM RADIOSURGERY

Gamma Knife Radiosurgery

The gamma knife is a dedicated radiosurgery machine, invented by Lars Leksell and his colleagues in 1968, in Sweden. Current gamma knife

Disclosures: The author has nothing to disclose.
Department of Neurological Surgery, University of Florida, PO Box 100265, MBI, Gainesville, FL 32610, USA
E-mail address: friedman@neurosurgery.ufl.edu

Neurosurg Clin N Am 24 (2013) 561–574
http://dx.doi.org/10.1016/j.nec.2013.05.002

equipment contains 192 cobalt-60 sources, held in a hemispherical array. These sources emit high-energy photons (called gamma rays). Each source creates an independent beam path through normal brain to the radiosurgery target. All of the beams coincide at the target, delivering a high dose of radiation, but each individual beam path has a small dose, creating a steep dose gradient, with little risk to normal tissue.

Steiner pioneered gamma knife radiosurgery for AVMs and has published multiple reports.[6–9] He reported 1-year occlusion rates ranging from 33.7% to 39.5% and 2-year occlusion rates ranging from 79% to 86.5%. However, these results were optimized by retrospectively selecting patients who received a high treatment dose. For example, in one report he stated that, "…a large majority of patients received at least 20–25 Gy of radiation. Of the 248 patients treated before 1984, the treatment specification placed 188 in this group."[10] The reported thrombosis rates in this article only applied to these 188 patients (76% of the total series).

Yamamoto and colleagues[11] reported on 25 Japanese patients treated on the gamma unit in Stockholm, but followed in Japan. The 2-year thrombosis rate in those AVMs that were completely covered by the radiosurgical field was 64%. One patient had complete thrombosis at 3-year angiography and an additional patient had complete thrombosis at 5-year angiography, for a total cure rate of 73%. In another article,[12] these investigators reported angiographic cures in 6 of 9 (67%) children treated in Stockholm or Buenos Aires and followed in Japan. Yamamoto and colleagues[13] reviewed the long-term follow-up results of a group of 40 Japanese patients undergoing gamma knife radiosurgery for AVMs in 3 different countries (Argentina, Sweden, and the United States). In this group of patients, the mean lesion volume was only 3.7 cm^3. Twenty-six patients (65%) were subsequently found to have angiographically confirmed nidus obliteration at 1 to 5 years after radiosurgery.

Kemeny and colleagues[14] reported on 52 patients with AVMs treated with gamma knife radiosurgery. They all received 25 Gy to the 50% isodose line. At 1 year, 16 patients (31%) had complete thrombosis and 10 patients (19%) had almost complete thrombosis. The results were better in younger patients and in patients with laterally located AVMs. There was no difference in outcome between small (<2 cm^3), medium (2–3 cm^3), and large (>3 cm^3) AVMs.

Lunsford and colleagues[15] reported on 227 patients with AVMs treated with gamma knife radiosurgery. The mean dose delivered to the AVM margin was 21.2 Gy. Multiple isocenters were used in 48% of the patients. Seventeen patients underwent 1-year angiography, which confirmed complete thrombosis in 76.5%. As indicated in the article, "this rate may be spurious since many of these patients were selected for angiography because their magnetic resonance (MR) image had suggested obliteration." Among 75 patients who were followed for at least 2 years, 2-year angiography was performed in only 46 (61%). Complete obliteration was confirmed in 37 of the 46 (80%). This thrombosis rate strongly correlated with AVM size, as follows: less than 1 cm^3, 100%; 1 to 4 cm^3, 85%; 4 to 10 cm^3, 58%. This group also reported on a group of 65 operable AVMs treated with radiosurgery.[16] Of 32 patients who subsequently underwent follow-up angiography, 84% showed complete thrombosis. In a later publication from this group, Pollock and colleagues[17] reported on 313 patients with AVMs. An angiographic cure rate of 61% was achieved.

Karlsson and colleagues[18] reported on 945 AVMs treated in Stockholm between 1970 and 1990 with the gamma knife. The overall occlusion rate was 56%. Shin and Maruyama[19] reported on 400 cases treated with gamma knife radiosurgery. They reported a 72% obliteration rate at 3 years after treatment. Other groups have reported on gamma knife radiosurgery results for specific sites like brainstem,[20,21] motor cortex,[22] or basal ganglia,[23] or in groups like children.[24]

Particle Beam (Proton or Helium) Radiosurgery

Particle beam radiosurgery facilities use cyclotron-like devices to accelerate subatomic particles to very high speeds before aiming them at patients. They have a unique physical property, called the Bragg peak effect, which results in most of the beam's energy being deposited at a predictable depth in tissue, with little exit dose. This property is theoretically ideal for radiosurgery but its usefulness has been limited by the need to spread out the Bragg peak to fit anatomic lesions, restrictions in beam number compared with gamma knife or linear accelerator systems, and the high cost of the facilities needed for such systems.

Kjellberg and colleagues[25–27] published multiple reports on the use of Bragg peak proton particle radiosurgery for AVMs. Their New England Journal of Medicine article in 1983 provided details on long-term follow-up of their first 75 patients.[28] It includes a well-known diagram of doses versus complications. However, only 20% of these patients had complete nidus obliteration on follow-up angiography. Seifert and colleagues[29] reported on 63 patients referred to the United States for Bragg peak proton beam therapy and followed in

Europe. Complete nidus obliteration was only seen in 10 patients (15.9%). Several patients had radiation-induced side effects.

In contrast, Steinberg and colleagues,[30] in an analysis of 86 AVMs treated with a helium particle beam radiosurgical system, reported a 29% 1 year thrombosis, 70% 2 year thrombosis, and 92% 3 year thrombosis rate. The best results were obtained with small lesions and high doses. At first a treatment dose of 34.6 Gy was used but a higher than expected neurologic complication rate (20% for the series) led to lower doses (7.7–19.2 Gy). No patients treated with the lower dose range had complications.

Linear Accelerator Radiosurgery

Linear accelerators are devices that use microwave energy to accelerate electrons to very high speeds. The energetic electrons collide with a heavy metal alloy in the head of the machine. Most of the collision energy is lost as heat, but a small percentage results in high-energy photon radiation (called x-rays because they are electronically produced). These photons are virtually identical to those produced by the spontaneous decay of radioactive cobalt in the gamma knife. They are collimated and focused on the radiosurgical target. Linear accelerator systems rotate the beam around the patient, from many different angles, to create the hundreds-of-beams approach used by the gamma knife to provide high doses at the target but low doses to normal tissues.

Betti pioneered linear accelerator radiosurgery and reported on the results of 66 AVMs treated with a linear accelerator radiosurgical system.[31–33] Doses of no more than 40 Gy were used in 80% of patients. He found a 66% 2-year thrombosis rate. The percentage of cured patients was highest when the entire malformation was included in the 75% isodose line (96%) or the maximum diameter of the lesion was less than 12 mm (81%).

Colombo and colleagues[34] reported on 97 patients with AVMs treated with a linear accelerator system. Doses from 18.7 to 40 Gy were delivered in 1 or 2 sessions. Of 56 patients who were followed for longer than 1 year, 50 underwent 12-month follow-up angiography. In 26 patients (52%), complete thrombosis was shown. Fifteen of 20 patients (75%) undergoing 2-year angiography had complete thrombosis. He reported a definite relationship between AVM size and thrombosis rate, as follows: lesions less than 15 mm in diameter had a 1 year obliteration rate of 76% and a 2 year rate of 90%. Lesions 15 to 25 mm in diameter had a 1-year thrombosis rate of 37.5% and a 2-year rate of 80%. Lesions greater than 25 mm in diameter had a 1-year thrombosis rate of 11% and a 2-year rate of 40%. In a later report, Colombo and colleagues[35] reported follow-up on 180 radiosurgically treated AVMs. The 1-year thrombosis rate was 46%, and the 2-year rate was 80%.

Souhami and colleagues[36] reported on 33 AVMs treated with a linear accelerator system. The prescribed dose at isocenter varied from 50 to 55 Gy. A complete obliteration rate of 38% was seen on 1-year angiography. For patients whose arteriovenous malformation nidus was covered by a minimum dose of 25 Gy, the total obliteration rate was 61.5%, whereas none of the patients who had received less than 25 Gy at the edge of the nidus obtained a total obliteration.

Loeffler and colleagues[37] reported on 16 AVMs treated with a linear accelerator system. The peripheral prescribed dose was 15 to 25 Gy, typically to the 80% to 90% line. The total obliteration rate was 5 of 11 (45%) at 1 year and 8 of 11 (73%) at 2 years after treatment.

Engenhart and colleagues[38] reported on the treatment of 212 patients in Heidelberg. "Above a threshold dose of 18 Gy, the obliteration rate was 72%. Radiation induced late complications were seen in 4.3%."

Schlienger and colleagues[39] reported on 169 patients treated in Paris. The overall obliteration rate was 64%. Success rates were higher in smaller lesions, in lesions not embolized, in lesions treated with higher doses, and lesions treated with 1 isocenter. Two patients experienced radiation-induced side effects.

Andrade-Souza and colleagues[40] reported on 38 rolandic area AVMs treated in Toronto. Complete nidus obliteration was seen in 60.5%. Two patients experienced radiation-induced side effects.

Friedman and colleagues[41–45] published multiple reports on the University of Florida experience with radiosurgery for AVMs. They documented occlusion rates of 80% for lesions less than 10 cm^3 in volume, with radiation-induced complications in the 2% range. Factors favoring occlusion include small AVM size, low Spetzler-Martin score, high peripheral radiation dose, and compact nidus morphology. Detailed dosimetric analysis suggested that 12 Gy volume and eloquent location correlated with transient radiation-induced complications.

RESULTS OF AVM RADIOSURGERY AT THE UNIVERSITY OF FLORIDA

Between 5/18/88 and 2/5/13, 699 AVMs were treated on the University of Florida radiosurgery system. There were 350 men and 349 women in the series. The mean age was 39 years (range 4–85 years). Patients presented with hemorrhage (225), seizure (264), headache/incidental finding (232), and progressive neurologic deficit (33). Thirty-eight patients had undergone prior subtotal microsurgical AVM excision. Fifty-five patients had undergone at least 1 embolization procedure. Patients were screened with a vascular neurosurgeon before consideration of radiosurgery.

The median lesion volume was 6.7 cm^3 (0.1–80 cm^3). The treatment volume was determined in all cases by performing a computerized dose volume histogram of the treatment isodose shell (which was constructed to conform closely to the AVM nidus). Lesion volumes were stratified as follows: A, less than 1 cm^3; B, 1 to 4 cm^3; C, 4 to 10 cm^3; D, greater than 10 cm^3. Spetzler-Martin grades were distributed as follows: grade I, 41 patients; grade II, 229 patients; grade III, 291 patients; and grade IV, 118 patients. The median radiation dose to the periphery of the lesion was 17.5 Gy (range 7.5–25 Gy). This treatment dose was delivered to the 80% isodose line when single isocenter plans were used, and to the 70% line when multiple isocenters were used. Three-hundred and eleven patients were treated with a single isocenter, 96 patients with 2 isocenters, 81 patients with 3 isocenters, 53 patients with 4 isocenters, and 143 patients with 5 isocenters or more.

Mean follow-up duration for the AVM group was 33 months (2–166 months). Follow-up generally consists of clinical examination and MR imaging (MRI) scanning at 1-year intervals after treatment, unless clinical symptoms indicated more frequent follow-up. When possible, follow-up is performed in Gainesville, Florida, otherwise scan and examination results are forwarded by the patient's local physician.

At first, all patients were asked to undergo angiography at yearly intervals, regardless of the MRI findings. After the first 50 patients were treated, it was decided to defer angiography until MRI/MR angiography strongly suggested complete thrombosis. Furthermore, if complete thrombosis was not identified 3 years after radiosurgery, repeat radiosurgery was undertaken in an effort to obliterate any remaining nidus (discussed later).

An angiographic cure required that no nidus or shunting remain on the study, as interpreted by a neuroradiologist and the treating neurosurgeon. Of the 192 follow-up angiograms performed to date, 147 (77%) have shown complete AVM obliteration. Using this traditional method of reporting, the following angiographic cure rates were seen in the various size categories: A, 93%; B, 86%; C, 83%; D, 53%. However, angiographic success rates can be misleadingly high, because

angiography may not be done if MRI shows residual nidus. If angiography or MRI follow-up results at 3 years are accepted, the following results are seen in 367 patients: A, 93%; B, 83%; C, 63%; D, 35%. In addition, if radiosurgical retreatments are included (which can salvage several initial failures, as discussed later), the patient success rates are as follows: A, 100%; B, 93%; C, 84%; D, 75%.

WHY DOES RADIOSURGERY FAIL?

In an effort to clarify the causes of radiosurgical failure, we[42] examined 36 patients who underwent repeat radiosurgery after an initial failure to obliterate their AVMs and compared them with 72 patients who were cured during the same time period. An image fusion methodology was used to fuse the treatment plan created at the first treatment to the computed tomography (CT) scan obtained at the time of retreatment. Two patients were excluded from the targeting error analysis because the nidus was too small to visualize on CT. Of the remaining 34 patients in whom the original treatment failed, 9 (26%) had a partial targeting error at the time of the first treatment.

The retreatment group had statistically significantly higher Spetzler-Martin grade, larger AVM size, and lower treatment dose compared with the group of patients who were cured. Statistical analysis also showed that patients treated with a peripheral dose of less than 15 Gy had a higher failure rate. In addition, patients with AVM volumes greater than 10 cm^3 had a higher failure rate.

Other radiosurgery groups have also published analyses designed to identify factors that might predict radiosurgical success or failure. Pollock and colleagues[17] found that the following factors predicted success: low AVM volume, few draining veins, young age, and superficial location. Prior embolization of the AVM was a negative predictor. This group also published a review of 45 patients who underwent repeat radiosurgical treatment after an initial treatment failed to obliterate their AVMs.[46] In this study, causes of radiosurgical failure were identified as follows: in 5 patients (11%), the entire AVM was not visualized secondary to incomplete angiography (2 vessels instead of 4 vessels) or inadequate angiographic technique (failure to perform superselective angiography). In 3 patients (7%), the AVM recanalized after previous embolization. In 4 patients (9%), the AVM nidus reexpanded after resorption of a prior hematoma that had compressed the vessels within the nidus. In 21 patients (46%), the three-dimensional shape of the AVM nidus was not appreciated secondary to reliance on biplanar angiography alone. In the remaining patients, a definite cause for failure could not be determined. The investigators thought that the AVMs in these patients had some form of radiobiological resistance; that is, failure to be obliterated despite proper planning and adequate dose delivery. In an earlier analysis by the same group,[47] the dose to the periphery (D_{min}) of the target was found to be the most significant predictor of success. In that analysis, neither volume nor maximum dose was predictive. Problems defining the complete AVM nidus were cited as significant limitations to successful AVM obliteration.

The Stockholm group published an analysis designed to define predictive factors for radiosurgical obliteration of AVMs.[48] Analyzing a 945-patient subset of the 1319 patients with AVMs treated with the gamma knife from 1970 to 1990, they again identified peripheral dose as the most significant predictive factor. The higher the minimum dose, the higher the obliteration rate, up to 25 Gy. The obliteration rate in the 268 cases that received this minimum dose (25 Gy) was 81%. High average dose and low AVM volume also predicted success. A high average dose shortened the latency to AVM obliteration. They proposed that the product of the cubed root of the AVM volume and the peripheral dose (the K index) would serve as a good combined predictor of success and found that a K index of 27 was optimal. Obliteration rates increased with increasing K values up to 27, beyond which no further improvement was observed.

Yamamoto and colleagues[13] reviewed the long-term follow-up results of a group of 40 Japanese patients undergoing gamma knife radiosurgery for AVMs in 3 different countries (Argentina, Sweden, and the United States). In this group of patients, the mean lesion volume was only 3.7 cm^3. Twenty-six patients (65%) were subsequently found to have angiographically confirmed nidus obliteration at 1 to 5 years after radiosurgery. Thirteen (32.5%) patients failed radiosurgery based on follow-up angiogram at 3 to 7 years after treatment. In their retrospective analysis, they discovered that the nidus had only partially been covered at the time of the first treatment in 6 of the 13 (46%) patients who subsequently failed.

The importance of targeting error as a cause for radiosurgical failure merits brief discussion. In the Pittsburgh series, 67% of all failures were attributed to targeting error resulting from inadequate imaging or obscuration of the AVM nidus by a hematoma. In Yamamoto's analysis,[13] targeting error was responsible for 46% of all failures. A similar analysis by Gallina and colleagues[49] attributed 10 of 17 (59%) AVM radiosurgery failures to inadequate targeting. In our experience,[42] targeting error was also an important cause of failure, accounting for 26% of failures, which may support the importance of using a three-dimensional database, such as contrast-enhanced CT or MR angiography, for targeting, as opposed to stereotactic angiography alone.

Zipfel and colleagues[50] explored the effect of AVM morphology on radiosurgical success. In 268 patients, diffuse nidus morphology and neovascularity were statistically significant predictors of failure. Meder and colleagues,[51] in an earlier study, also documented the importance of angioarchitecture.

Pollock and Flickinger[52,53] developed an AVM grading system that accurately predicts the chances of an excellent outcome (meaning occlusion and no radiation-induced side effects) after radiosurgery. In a multivariate analysis of 220 patients, 5 variables related to excellent outcome: AVM volume, patient age, AVM location, previous embolization, and number of draining veins. Further analysis permitted the removal of 2 variables (embolization and draining veins), yielding the following predictive equation: AVM score = 0.1 (AVM volume) + 0.02 (patient age in years) + 0.3 (location of lesion). Locations scores are: frontal or temporal = 0; parietal, occipital, intraventricular, corpus callosum, cerebellar = 1; basal ganglia, thalamic, brainstem = 2. All patients with an AVM score less than 1 had an excellent outcome, compared with only 39% of patients with a score higher than 2. The Spetzler-Martin score and the K index did not correlate with excellent outcome. This group subsequently showed that the AVM score also predicted the chance of a worsened Modified Rankin Scale score after radiosurgical treatment.[54] Andrade-Souza and colleagues[55] verified the predictive value of the AVM score in 136 patients treated with linear accelerator–based radiosurgery. The University of Florida series was analyzed with this technique and we also confirmed its validity.[56]

HEMORRHAGE AFTER RADIOSURGERY

There are significant pitfalls to be avoided in the analysis of hemorrhage risk after radiosurgery. First, because radiosurgery is usually successful, a large number of patients are eliminated from the at-risk pool during the first and second years after radiosurgery. Failure to adequately account for this leads to the false impression that the smaller number of hemorrhages occurring greater than 1 year after treatment are caused by some protective effect. The decreasing number of hemorrhages is statistically caused by the decreasing number of patients at risk. Second, because a significant number of patients present with hemorrhage in any radiosurgery series, and because these patients may have an increased risk of hemorrhage for the first 6 months after hemorrhage, the incidence of bleeding in the first 6 months after treatment may seem, in some series, to be increased. This observation is likely not a direct effect of radiosurgery, but rather a reflection of the inclusion of this group of patients with a higher-than-normal risk of hemorrhage. Series that treat a large percentage of patients presenting with hemorrhage (as opposed to seizures or headache) might for this reason be expected to have an increased hemorrhage rate during the first 6 months after treatment. Third, and most important, the incidence of hemorrhage in patients with AVMs is small, which means that the effect of a slight alteration in the number of hemorrhages over a given period of time may, without the benefit of statistical analysis, significantly skew the conclusions in this type of analysis. Assuming a constant baseline AVM hemorrhage rate of 3 per 100 person-years follow-up (or 3% per year) in untreated patients, 726 person-years of follow-up would be required to have a 95% chance of detecting a reduction in the hemorrhage rate to 1 per 100 person-years of follow-up (or 1% per year) in treated patients at a 0.05 significance level. Given the high cure rate of radiosurgery, a large number (thousands) of patients treated would be needed to generate a sufficient number of patient follow-up years in years 2, 3, 4, and so forth, in order to yield statistically valid information. These factors must be kept in mind when interpreting some of the articles discussed later. Any attempt to elucidate the question of AVM bleeding after radiosurgery without benefit of detailed statistics must be viewed with skepticism.

The issue of AVM hemorrhage after radiosurgical treatment was first discussed by investigators using particle beam methodology. Kjellberg and colleagues[28] initially reported 2 deaths from hemorrhage in the first year after treatment of their first 75 patients. In a subsequent report of 389 patients followed for at least 2 years, 8 had succumbed from hemorrhage in the first 2 years after treatment.[25] Only 1 had died thereafter, for a 0.27% mortality in those patients greater than 2 years after treatment. At first, these investigators suggested that only those patients presenting with hemorrhage were at risk for subsequent lethal rebleeding. However, later reports document fatal hemorrhage in patients presenting with seizure only. It should be emphasized that these investigators reported a total hemorrhage rate of 2.4% per year (lethal and nonlethal) for those patients more than 2 years out from treatment. Whether this differs from the natural history of the disease is debatable.

Other particle beam proponents have also addressed the hemorrhage question. Steinberg and colleagues[30] reported 10 hemorrhages (2 fatal), occurring between 4 and 34 months after radiosurgical treatment, in a series of 86 patients (12%). Two of these patients had hemorrhages in the third year after treatment, suggesting no protective effect unless complete obliteration was achieved. Seifert and colleagues[29] analyzed a series of 68 patients treated with proton beam therapy in the United States. Eighteen patients deteriorated neurologically. Five of them had hemorrhages, of which 2 were fatal.

Gamma knife radiosurgeons have studied this question as well. Lunsford and colleagues,[15] in an initial report on AVM treatment with the Pittsburgh gamma knife, noted that 10 patients (4%) in a series of 227 patients had experienced hemorrhage. Two of these patients died. Pollock and colleagues,[16] in a study of 65 patients with operable AVMs, noted that 5 patients had a hemorrhage (7.7%), all within 8 months of radiosurgery. Two of these patients died. Steiner and colleagues[57] statistically analyzed bleeding in 247 consecutive AVM cases. The Kaplan-Meier approach showed a risk of nearly 3.7% per year until 5 years after radiosurgery, at which point a plateau was reached. This plateau was thought to be caused by the small number of data points for that time period and not to indicate any protective effect. Karlsson and colleagues[58] reported an analysis of bleeding in 1565 patients treated with the Stockholm gamma knife. They thought that the risk of hemorrhage was decreased, even with incomplete obliteration. They also reported that increasing age and increasing AVM volume correlated with an increased risk of hemorrhage.

Betti and colleagues,[31] in their pioneering report on linear accelerator radiosurgery for AVMs, documented hemorrhage in 5 of 66 (8%) of their patients. These hemorrhages occurred at 12, 18, 22, 25, and 29 months after treatment. All had a prior history of hemorrhage. Two of these patients died. Colombo and colleagues[35] also reported a detailed analysis of 180 patients. Fifteen patients had hemorrhages and 5 of them succumbed. In cases in which the AVM nidus was totally irradiated, the bleeding risk decreased from 4.8% during the first 6 months to 0% starting from the 12th month of follow-up. In partially irradiated cases, the bleeding risk increased from 4% in the first 6 months to 10% from the sixth to the 18th month and then down to 5.5% from the 18th to the 24th month. No bleeding was observed thereafter.

Our analysis of this issue[59] did not reveal any postradiosurgical alteration in bleeding risk from the 3% to 4% per year expected based on natural history. A similar study by the Pittsburgh group confirmed that "stereotactic radiosurgery was not associated with a significant change in the hemorrhage rate of AVMs during the latency interval before obliteration."[60]

As discussed earlier, Karlsson and colleagues[58] reported an increased risk of AVM hemorrhage with increasing AVM size. Colombo and colleagues[61] found a higher incidence in subtotally irradiated AVMs, most of which were presumably large lesions. He also reported a statistically increased risk in patients treated more inhomogeneously (to a lower isodose line). In a subsequent article,[35] his group attributed this observation to the earlier thrombosis of the portion of the AVM receiving the highest dose of radiation, with shunting of blood into the remaining nidus, increasing the risk of hemorrhage.

In our series, a correlation between AVM volume and the risk of hemorrhage was also found. Ten of the 12 AVMs that bled were greater than 10 cm^3 in volume. In addition, the correlation of hemorrhage with low dose and low isodose line treated was likely caused by the deliberate use of low doses and multiple isocenter treatments (to low isodose lines) in large AVMs. Of equal importance are those factors that did not statistically correlate with bleeding risk. In this study, neither age nor history of prior hemorrhage correlated with the incidence of hemorrhage.

Pollock and colleagues[62] found a significant correlation between the incidence of postradiosurgical hemorrhage and presence of an unsecured proximal aneurysm, and recommended that such aneurysms be obliterated before radiosurgery. The same group also studied factors associated with bleeding risk of AVMs and found 3 AVM characteristics to predict greater hemorrhage risk: (1) history of prior bleed, (2) presence of a single draining vein, and (3) diffuse AVM morphology. Nataf and colleagues[63] analyzed bleeding after radiosurgery for 756 patients with AVMs. The actuarial hemorrhage rate was 3.08% per year per patient. It increased from 1.66% the first year to 3.87% in the 5th year after radiosurgery, but was never statistically different from the rate before radiosurgery. Intranidal aneurysms, complete coverage, and minimum dose correlated with the risk of hemorrhage.

Maruyama and colleagues[64] performed a retrospective observational study of 500 patients. Compared with the period between diagnosis and radiosurgery, the risk of hemorrhage decreased by 54% during the latency period, and by 88% after obliteration. The risk of hemorrhage was not eliminated by angiographic obliteration. Other investigators have also reported rare cases of AVM bleeding after documented angiographic obliteration.

In summary, the major drawback of radiosurgical AVM treatment is the risk of bleeding during the latent period (typically 2 years) between treatment and AVM thrombosis. Most studies suggest that the natural history risk of hemorrhage remains unchanged until thrombosis. Some suggest that the bleeding risk decreases, even before thrombosis. Even after thrombosis occurs, there seems to be a small risk of continued hemorrhage. At this time, only surgery can immediately and completely eliminate the risk of AVM bleeding.

RADIATION-INDUCED COMPLICATIONS

Acute complications are rare after AVM radiosurgery. Several investigators have reported that radiosurgery can acutely exacerbate seizure activity. Others have reported nausea, vomiting, and headache occasionally occurring after radiosurgical treatment.[65]

Delayed radiation-induced complications have been reported by all groups performing radiosurgery. In 1984, Steiner[7] reported symptomatic radiation necrosis in approximately 3% of his patients. Statham and colleagues[66] described one patient who developed radiation necrosis 13 months after gamma knife radiosurgery of a 5.3-cm^3 AVM with 25 Gy to the margin. In 1991, Lunsford and colleagues[15] reported that 10 patients in the Pittsburgh series (4.4%) developed new neurologic deficits thought to be secondary to radiation injury. Symptoms were location dependent and developed between 4 and 18 months after treatment. All patients were treated with steroids and all improved. Only 2 patients were reported to have residual deficits that seemed permanent. In this early analysis, the radiation dose and isodose line treated did not correlate with incidence of complication. As he noted, the failure of correlation of dose and complications likely related to the doses having been selected to be below Flickinger's[67–69] computed 3% risk line, which is a mathematically derived line that prescribes low doses for large lesions, and underpins the well-established correlation between increasing radiosurgical target volume and increasing incidence of radiation necrosis.

Flickinger and colleagues[70] published an analysis of complications from AVM radiosurgery that emphasizes the importance of lesion location and dose. The analysis, which includes outcome data from 332 Pittsburgh gamma knife AVM radiosurgery cases from 1987 to 1994, found that 30 patients (9%) developed some symptomatic postradiosurgery sequelae (any neurologic problem including headache). Symptoms resolved in 58% of these patients within 27 months. The statistical likelihood of having a transient versus a permanent deficit was dose dependent, with a difference noted at a peripheral dose of 20 Gy (D_{min}). When D_{min} was less than 20 Gy, 89% of patients who developed deficits experienced complete resolution of their symptoms, whereas only 36% of patients receiving minimum target doses greater than 20 Gy fully recovered. The 7-year actuarial rate for developing a permanent radiation-induced neurologic deficit was 3.8%. The relative risks for various lesion locations were compared, and a postradiosurgery injury expression (PIE) score was assigned to various brain locations. In general, deep locations had high PIE scores, indicating a high risk of radiation-induced complications. Multivariate statistical analysis identified only PIE location score and 12-Gy volume as significant predictors of radiation-induced symptomatic sequelae. Variables analyzed but found not to be significant predictors of complications included prior neurologic deficit, prior hemorrhage, use of MRI-enhanced treatment planning, prescription isodose line, and number of isocenters. The same group has published numerous other articles documenting the value of this approach.[71–73]

The Stockholm group published an analysis of factors associated with complications following AVM radiosurgery.[48] Their report confirms the predictive importance of AVM location and dose. A history of prior hemorrhage was associated with a low risk of complications in their series, and prior radiation was associated with a high risk of complications.

Steinberg and colleagues[30] reported a correlation between lesion size, lesion dose, and complications. Their initial treatment dose of 34.6 Gy led to a high complication rate. Patients were subsequently treated with a lower dose and had no radiation-induced complications. In an earlier report on 75 patients with AVMs treated with helium particles, at a dose of 45 Gy, 7 of 75 patients (11%) experienced radiation-induced complications.[74]

Kjellberg and colleagues[28] and Kjellberg and Abbe,[75] using a compilation of animal and clinical data, constructed a series of log-log lines, relating prescribed dose and lesion diameter. Their 1% isorisk line is similar to Flickinger's[67–69] mathematically derived 3% risk line.

In Colombo and colleagues'[35] series, 9 of 180 (5%) patients experienced symptomatic radiation-induced complications. Four (2.2%) were permanent. Loeffler and colleagues[76] reported that 1 of

21 patients with AVMs developed a similar problem, which responded well to steroids. Souhami and colleagues[36] reported severe side effects in 2 of 33 (6%) patients. Marks and colleagues[77] reviewed 6 radiosurgical series and found a 9% overall incidence of clinically significant radiation reactions. Seven of 23 cases received doses below Kjellberg's 1% risk line.

Chen and colleagues[78] reported a case of aggressive, recurrent cerebral necrosis leading to death, despite surgical intervention. Others have suggested that occlusive hyperemia (caused by venous thrombosis), not radiation necrosis, may be responsible for radiation-induced side effects.

At the University of Florida, 12 patients (2.5%) have sustained permanent radiation-induced side effects. Fifteen (3%) have sustained transient side effects. A detailed analysis of dosimetric factors revealed that 12-Gy volume and eloquent brain location correlated with transient complications. No factor predicted permanent complications. We reported 1 case of symptomatic radiation-induced hemiparesis successfully treated with hyperbaric oxygen.[79]

VERY-LATE-ONSET COMPLICATIONS

Yamamoto and colleagues[13,80–83] have published a series of articles describing radiation-related adverse effects observed on late neuroimaging after AVM radiosurgery. In their study of 53 patients status post gamma knife AVM radiosurgery, MRI was performed up to 10 years after treatment. In this series, of the 5 patients (9.4%) who developed delayed neurologic symptoms, 3 presented at least 5 years after treatment. One patient with a midbrain AVM developed a hemi-Parkinson syndrome 5.5 years after radiosurgery. Another patient developed gradual visual field narrowing accompanied by signs of increased intracranial pressure 7 years after treatment: MRI revealed a large cyst in the left parieto-occipital lobe at the site of the irradiated AVM, and surgery was required. The third patient presented 7 years after treatment with hemiparesis caused by a diffuse white matter necrotic lesion.

Also concerning was the late development of 4 additional asymptomatic radiological abnormalities. One middle cerebral artery stenosis of the M1 segment was detected 3 years after radiation treatment. A dural arteriovenous fistula developed 7 years after treatment, and 2 delayed cysts had formed at 5 and 10 years following treatment.

The lesion volumes and treatment doses used in this series were not unusual (median volume 1.5 cm^3, mean peripheral target dose 21.5 Gy), and careful examination of the complicated cases reveals no obvious deviation from standard radiosurgical practice. Meticulous radiological follow-up may explain some of these unusual findings. Perhaps such abnormalities are not rare, but (especially in the cases of asymptomatic patients) are simply going undetected.

Kihlstrom and colleagues[84] also reported a series of late radiological abnormalities after AVM radiosurgery. MRI scans and follow-up angiography were performed on 18 patients at a mean interval of 14 years (8–23 years) after radiosurgical treatment. All patients had previous angiographic documentation of AVM obliteration, and all were clinically asymptomatic. Radiological findings included cyst formation at the previous AVM site in 5 patients (28%), contrast enhancement at the former lesion site (without AVM recanalization) in 11 patients (61%), and increased T2 MR signal at the former lesion site in 3 patients (17%). In this series (unlike the case reported by Yamamoto) none of the observed cysts exceeded 2 cm in diameter, all were confined to the volume of the previous AVM nidus, and none caused any mass effect. Because treatment doses used in this study were higher than those currently administered, it is difficult to predict whether similar findings will be reproduced in more recent patient series. The absence of clinical symptoms in these patients may indicate that such late radiographic abnormalities are of limited clinical importance.

Hara and colleagues[85] also reported 2 cases of delayed cyst formation after AVM radiosurgery.

SALVAGE RETREATMENT OF FAILED AVM RADIOSURGERY

Several groups have reported on the use of repeat radiosurgery as a salvage technique after failed AVM radiosurgery. The Stockholm radiosurgery group analyzed 101 cases of such salvage retreatment.[86] Obliteration was achieved in 62% of these cases, a rate almost identical to that currently reported by this group for primary AVM radiosurgery. The complication rate was 14%, which was significantly higher than that currently reported by this group for primary radiosurgery. The annual risk of hemorrhage during the first 2 posttreatment years was 1.8%, a value not statistically different from that associated with the natural history of this disease. In a more recent evaluation of 133 patients with an initial nidus volume of 9 cm^3 or more, the estimated obliteration rate was 62% following repeat treatment.[87] Four patients (3%) developed radiation-induced side effects and 5 others (4%) developed cystic changes.

Maesawa and Flickinger[88] reported on repeat radiosurgery in 41 patients. The estimated 2-year

obliteration rate was 71%. Two patients developed radiation-induced side effects.

Mirza-Aghazadeh and colleagues[89] reported on 12 retreatments using a linear accelerator system. Two-thirds were cured, with a radiation-induced complication rate of 13%. Raza and colleagues[90] reported on 14 retreatments. They achieved a complete obliteration rate of 35.7%.

Schlienger and colleagues[91] reported on 41 patients retreated in their Paris unit. The obliteration rate was 59.3%. They had a 9% complication rate. Foote and colleagues[92] reported on 52 patients retreated at the University of Florida. Sixty percent were obliterated on follow-up angiography, with no reported permanent radiation side effects. The current salvage rate at the University of Florida after retreatment is 70%.

In 2000, Pollock and colleagues[93] described an alternative retreatment approach that they called staged-volume arteriovenous malformation radiosurgery. The idea involves treating only part of the AVM nidus, then returning later (typically 6 months) and treating the other part. In 2006, Sirin and colleagues[94] reported on 37 patients who had undergone such therapy. The initial AVM volume averaged 24.9 cm^3. The median marginal dose was 16 Gy at both treatments. Of 14 patients followed for more than 36 months, 50% had total occlusion and 29% had near-total occlusion.

MULTIMODALITY AVM TREATMENT

When an AVM is amenable to safe microsurgical resection, this therapy is preferred because it offers immediate cure and elimination of hemorrhage risk. When the estimated morbidity of resection is excessive, radiosurgery offers a reasonable chance for delayed cure. However, some unresectable AVMs, by virtue of their large size, are not candidates for radiosurgery. These problematic lesions may be managed with presurgery or preradiosurgery embolization.

Before radiosurgery, the most important role of embolization is to reduce the size of the lesion. Potential secondary advantages of preradiosurgical embolization are that associated aneurysms may be treated, and high-flow arteriovenous fistulae (thought to be less sensitive to radiosurgery) may be identified and occluded.

Dawson and colleagues[95] reported on 7 patients with large AVMs who were treated with embolization followed by gamma knife radiosurgery. At 2-year follow-up, 2 AVMs were obliterated, and 2 others had a 98% reduction in volume. Lemme-Plaghos and colleagues[96] reported their results in 16 patients with high-grade AVMs who were treated with embolization and gamma knife radiosurgery.

Four cures (25%) were reported. Mathis and colleagues[97] reported on a series of patients with large AVMs (volume>10 cm^3) who were treated with embolization and radiosurgery. Of the 56 patients treated, 24 were included in their analysis and 12 were cured. Among the analyzed group, 2 patients (8%) experienced transient neurologic deficit after embolization, and 1 developed mild upper extremity weakness after radiosurgery. Recanalization of previously embolized, but not irradiated, regions of AVM nidus occurred in 3 patients. Guo and colleagues[98] reported on 46 patients treated with embolization and gamma knife radiosurgery. In 16 cases, collateral vessels developed that made subsequent delineation of the nidus for radiosurgery difficult. In addition, 9 patients had neurologic complications after embolization. Only 19 of 35 large AVMs were reduced in size enough to be subsequently treatable with radiosurgery.

A larger series of patients treated with a combination of embolization and linear accelerator radiosurgery was reported on by Gobin and colleagues.[99] Of the 125 AVMs treated with (usually multiple session) endovascular treatment, 14 (11%) were completely occluded with embolization alone. Ninety-six AVMs (77%) were reduced in size by embolization enough to be considered for radiosurgery. Of those who underwent postembolization radiosurgery, complete occlusion was achieved in 65%. Embolization resulted in a mortality of 1.6% and a morbidity rate of 12.8%. No complications were associated with radiosurgery in this series. The posttreatment AVM hemorrhage rate was 3% per year. Despite the use of cyanoacrylate (the current standard in durable embolic material), a 12% revascularization rate was observed.

Henkes and colleagues[100] reported on 64 patients treated with embolization and radiosurgery. Of 30 patients followed beyond the latency interval, 14 (43%) had angiographic cures. Zabel-du Bois and colleagues[101] reported on 50 patients treated with embolization and radiosurgery. The actuarial obliteration rate was 67% at 3 years. Small AVMs and low Spetzler-Martin scores had high obliteration rates.

Embolization is an excellent adjunct to open surgical resection of AVMs but its role in radiosurgery is less clear. At the University of Florida, we try to avoid combining embolization and radiosurgery. Embolization tends to convert a compact nidal target into multiple remaining islands of nidus, which are difficult to clearly identify and target. Embolic material tends to create artifact on CT and MRI, further reducing radiosurgical targeting ability. Embolic material can wash out, leading to recanalization after radiosurgery. In addition, embolization has a small but real risk of neurologic complications. For these reasons, we prefer to use radiosurgery, with repeat treatment if necessary, for large AVMs.

REFERENCES

1. Leksell L. The stereotaxic method and radiosurgery of the brain. Acta Chir Scand 1951;102:316–9.
2. Yamamoto M, Jimbo M, Ide M, et al. Gamma knife radiosurgery for cerebral arteriovenous malformations: an autopsy report focusing on irradiation-induced changes observed in nidus-unrelated arteries. Surg Neurol 1995;44:421–7.
3. Szeifert GT, Kemeny AA, Timperley WR, et al. The potential role of myofibroblasts in the obliteration of arteriovenous malformations after radiosurgery. Neurosurgery 1997;40:61–5.
4. Schneider BF, Eberhard DA, Steiner L. Histopathology of arteriovenous malformations after gamma knife radiosurgery. J Neurosurg 1997;87:352–7.
5. Chang SD, Shuster DL, Steinberg GK, et al. Stereotactic radiosurgery of arteriovenous malformations: pathologic changes in resected tissue. Clin Neuropathol 1997;16:111–6.
6. Steiner L. Radiosurgery in cerebral arteriovenous malformations. In: Fein JM, Flamm ES, editors. Cerebrovascular surgery, vol. 4. New York: Springer-Verlag; 1985. p. 1161–215.
7. Steiner L. Treatment of arteriovenous malformations by radiosurgery. In: Wilson CB, Stein BM, editors. Intracranial arteriovenous malformations. Baltimore: Williams & Wilkins; 1984. p. 295–313.
8. Steiner L, Leksell L, Forster DM, et al. Stereotactic radiosurgery in intracranial arteriovenous malformations. Acta Neurochir Suppl 1974;21:195–209.
9. Steiner L, Leksell L, Greitz T, et al. Stereotaxic radiosurgery for cerebral arteriovenous malformations. Report of a case. Acta Chir Scand 1972;138:459–64.
10. Lindquist C, Steiner L. Stereotactic radiosurgical treatment of malformations of the brain. In: Modern stereotactic neurosurgery. Boston: Martinus Nijhoff; 1988. p. 491–506.
11. Yamamoto M, Jimbo M, Kobayashi M, et al. Long-term results of radiosurgery for arteriovenous malformation: neurodiagnostic imaging and histological studies of angiographically confirmed nidus obliteration. Surg Neurol 1992;37:219–30.
12. Yamamoto M, Jimbo M, Ide M, et al. Long-term follow-up of radiosurgically treated arteriovenous malformations in children: report of nine cases. Surg Neurol 1992;38:95–100.
13. Yamamoto M, Jimbo M, Hara M, et al. Gamma knife radiosurgery for arteriovenous malformations: long-term follow-up results focusing on complications

occurring more than five years after irradiation. Neurosurgery 1996;38:906–14.

14. Kemeny AA, Dias PS, Forster D. Results of stereotactic radiosurgery of arteriovenous malformations: an analysis of 52 cases. J Neurol Neurosurg Psychiatr 1989;52:554–8.

15. Lunsford LD, Kondziolka D, Flickinger JC, et al. Stereotactic radiosurgery for arteriovenous malformations of the brain. J Neurosurg 1991;75: 512–24.

16. Pollock BE, Lunsford LD, Kondziolka D, et al. Patient outcomes after stereotactic radiosurgery for "operable" arteriovenous malformations. Neurosurgery 1994;35:1–8.

17. Pollock BE, Flickinger JC, Lunsford LD, et al. Factors associated with successful arteriovenous malformation radiosurgery. Neurosurgery 1998;42: 1239–44.

18. Karlsson B, Lindquist C, Steiner L. Prediction of obliteration after gamma knife surgery for cerebral arteriovenous malformations. Neurosurgery 1997; 40:425–30.

19. Shin M, Maruyama K, Kurita H, et al. Analysis of nidus obliteration rates after gamma knife surgery for arteriovenous malformations based on longterm follow-up data: the University of Tokyo experience. J Neurosurg 2004;101:18–24.

20. Maruyama K, Kondziolka D, Niranjan A, et al. Stereotactic radiosurgery for brainstem arteriovenous malformations: factors affecting outcome. J Neurosurg 2004;100:407–13.

21. Kurita H, Kawamoto S, Sasaki T, et al. Results of radiosurgery for brain stem arteriovenous malformations. J Neurol Neurosurg Psychiatr 2000;68: 563–70.

22. Hadjipanayis CG, Levy EI, Niranjan A, et al. Stereotactic radiosurgery for motor cortex region arteriovenous malformations. Neurosurgery 2001;48:70–7.

23. Pollock BE, Gorman DA, Brown PD. Radiosurgery for arteriovenous malformations of the basal ganglia, thalamus, and brainstem. J Neurosurg 2004;100:210–4.

24. Kiran NA, Kale SS, Vaishya S, et al. Gamma knife surgery for intracranial arteriovenous malformations in children: a retrospective study in 103 patients. J Neurosurg 2007;107:479–84.

25. Kjellberg RN. Stereotactic Bragg peak proton beam radiosurgery for cerebral arteriovenous malformations. Ann Clin Res 1986;18(Suppl 47): 17–9.

26. Kjellberg RN, Davis KR, Lyons S, et al. Bragg peak proton beam therapy for arteriovenous malformations of the brain. Clin Neurosurg 1983;31:248.

27. Kjellberg RN, Poletti CE, Roberson GH, et al. Bragg-peak proton beam treatment of arteriovenous malformation of the brain. Excerpta Med 1977;433:181–6.

28. Kjellberg RN, Hanamura T, Davis KR, et al. Bragg-peak proton-beam therapy for arteriovenous malformations of the brain. N Engl J Med 1983;309: 269–74.

29. Seifert V, Stolke D, Mehdorn HM, et al. Clinical and radiological evaluation of long-term results of stereotactic proton beam radiosurgery in patients with cerebral arteriovenous malformations. J Neurosurg 1994;81:683–9.

30. Steinberg GK, Fabrikant JI, Marks MP, et al. Stereotactic heavy-charged particle Bragg peak radiation for intracranial arteriovenous malformations. N Engl J Med 1990;323:96–101.

31. Betti OO, Munari C, Rosler R. Stereotactic radiosurgery with the linear accelerator: treatment of arteriovenous malformations. Neurosurgery 1989;24: 311–21.

32. Betti OO. Treatment of arteriovenous malformations with the linear accelerator. Appl Neurophysiol 1987;50:262.

33. Betti OO, Derechinsky VE. Hyperselective encephalic irradiation with a linear accelerator. Acta Neurochir Suppl 1984;33:385–90.

34. Colombo F, Benedetti A, Pozza F, et al. Linear accelerator radiosurgery of cerebral arteriovenous malformations. Neurosurgery 1989;24:833–40.

35. Colombo F, Pozza F, Chierego G, et al. Linear accelerator radiosurgery of cerebral arteriovenous malformations: an update. Neurosurgery 1994;34: 14–21.

36. Souhami L, Olivier A, Podgorsak EB, et al. Radiosurgery of cerebral arteriovenous malformations with the dynamic stereotactic irradiation. Int J Radiat Oncol Biol Phys 1990;19:775–82.

37. Loeffler JS, Alexander EI, Siddon RL, et al. Stereotactic radiosurgery for intracranial arteriovenous malformations using a standard linear accelerator. Int J Radiat Oncol Biol Phys 1989;17:673–7.

38. Engenhart R, Wowra B, Debus J, et al. The role of high-dose single fraction irradiation in small and large intracranial arteriovenous malformations. Int J Radiat Oncol Biol Phys 1994;30:521–9.

39. Schlienger M, Atlan D, Lefkopoulos D, et al. LINAC radiosurgery for cerebral arteriovenous malformations. Int J Radiat Oncol Biol Phys 2000;46:1135–42.

40. Andrade-Souza YM, Ramani M, Scora D, et al. Radiosurgical treatment for rolandic arteriovenous malformations. J Neurosurg 2006;105:689–97.

41. Friedman WA, Bova FJ, Bollampally S, et al. Analysis of factors predictive of success or complications in arteriovenous malformation radiosurgery. Neurosurgery 2003;52:296–307.

42. Ellis TL, Friedman WA, Bova FJ, et al. Analysis of treatment failure after radiosurgery for arteriovenous malformations. J Neurosurg 1998;89: 104–10.

43. Friedman WA, Bova FJ, Mendenhall W. Linear accelerator radiosurgery for arteriovenous malformations: the relationship of size to outcome. J Neurosurg 1995;82:180–9.

44. Friedman WA, Bova FJ. Radiosurgery for arteriovenous malformations. In: Salcman M, editor. Current Techniques in Radiosurgery. Philadelphia: Current Medicine; 1993. p. 11.1–4.

45. Friedman WA, Bova FJ. LINAC radiosurgery for arteriovenous malformations. J Neurosurg 1992; 77:832–41.

46. Pollock BE, Kondziolka D, Lunsford LD, et al. Repeat stereotactic radiosurgery of arteriovenous malformations: factors associated with incomplete obliteration. Neurosurgery 1996;38:318–24.

47. Flickinger JC, Pollock BE, Kondziolka D, et al. A dose-response analysis of arteriovenous malformation obliteration after radiosurgery. Int J Radiat Oncol Biol Phys 1996;36:873–9.

48. Karlsson B, Lax I, Soderman M. Factors influencing the risk for complications following gamma knife radiosurgery of cerebral arteriovenous malformations. Radiother Oncol 1997;43:275–80.

49. Gallina P, Merienne L, Meder JF, et al. Failure in radiosurgery treatment of cerebral arteriovenous malformations. Neurosurgery 1998;42:996–1002.

50. Zipfel GJ, Bradshaw P, Bova FJ, et al. Do the morphological characteristics of arteriovenous malformations affect the results of radiosurgery? J Neurosurg 2004;101:393–401.

51. Meder JF, Oppenheim C, Blustajn J, et al. Cerebral arteriovenous malformations: the value of radiologic parameters in predicting response to radiosurgery. AJNR Am J Neuroradiol 1997;18: 1473–83.

52. Pollock BE, Flickinger JC. A proposed radiosurgery-based grading system for arteriovenous malformations. J Neurosurg 2002;96:79–85.

53. Pollock BE, Gorman DA, Coffey RJ. Patient outcomes after arteriovenous malformation radiosurgical management: results based on a 5- to 14-year follow-up study. Neurosurgery 2003;52: 1291–6.

54. Pollock BE, Brown RD. Use of the Modified Rankin Scale to assess outcome after arteriovenous malformation radiosurgery. Neurology 2006;67: 1630–4.

55. Andrade-Souza YM, Zadeh G, Ramani M, et al. Testing the radiosurgery-based arteriovenous malformation score and the modified Spetzler-Martin grading system to predict radiosurgical outcome. J Neurosurg 2005;103:642–8.

56. Raffa SJ, Chi YY, Bova FJ, et al. Validation of the radiosurgery-based arteriovenous malformation score in a large linear accelerator radiosurgery experience. J Neurosurg 2009;111:832–9.

57. Steiner L, Lindquist C, Adler JR, et al. Clinical outcome of radiosurgery for cerebral arteriovenous malformations. J Neurosurg 1992;77:1–8.

58. Karlsson B, Lax I, Soderman M. Risk for hemorrhage during the 2-year latency period following gamma knife radiosurgery for arteriovenous malformations. Int J Radiat Oncol Biol Phys 2001;49: 1045–51.

59. Friedman WA, Blatt DL, Bova FJ, et al. The risk of hemorrhage after radiosurgery for arteriovenous malformations. J Neurosurg 1996;84:912–9.

60. Pollock BE, Flickinger JC, Lunsford LD, et al. Hemorrhage risk after stereotactic radiosurgery of cerebral arteriovenous malformations. Neurosurgery 1996;38:652–61.

61. Colombo F, Francescon P, Cora S, et al. Evaluation of linear accelerator radiosurgical techniques using biophysical parameters (NTCP and TCP). Int J Radiat Oncol Biol Phys 1995;31:617–28.

62. Pollock BE, Flickinger JC, Lunsford LD, et al. Factors that predict the bleeding risk of cerebral arteriovenous malformations. Stroke 1996; 27:1–6.

63. Nataf F, Ghossoub M, Schlienger M, et al. Bleeding after radiosurgery for cerebral arteriovenous malformations. Neurosurgery 2004;55:298–305.

64. Maruyama K, Kawahara N, Shin M, et al. The risk of hemorrhage after radiosurgery for cerebral arteriovenous malformations. N Engl J Med 2005;352: 146–53.

65. Alexander EI, Siddon RL, Loeffler JS. The acute onset of nausea and vomiting following stereotactic radiosurgery: correlation with total dose to area postrema. Surg Neurol 1989;32:40–4.

66. Statham P, Macpherson P, Johnston R, et al. Cerebral radiation necrosis complicating stereotactic radiosurgery for arteriovenous malformation. J Neurol Neurosurg Psychiatr 1990;53:476–9.

67. Flickinger JC, Lunsford LD, Wu A, et al. Predicted dose-volume isoeffect curves for stereotactic radiosurgery with the 60Co gamma unit. Acta Oncol 1991;30:363–7.

68. Flickinger JC, Steiner L. Radiosurgery and the double logistic product formula. Radiother Oncol 1990; 17:229–37.

69. Flickinger JC, Schell MC, Larson DA. Estimation of complications for linear accelerator radiosurgery with the integrated logistic formula. Int J Radiat Oncol Biol Phys 1990;19:143–8.

70. Flickinger JC, Kondziolka D, Pollock BE, et al. Complications from arteriovenous malformation radiosurgery: multivariate analysis and risk modeling. Int J Radiat Oncol Biol Phys 1997;38:485–90.

71. Flickinger JC, Kondziolka D, Lunsford LD, et al. Development of a model to predict permanent symptomatic postradiosurgery injury for arteriovenous

malformation patients. Int J Radiat Oncol Biol Phys 2000;46:1143–8.

72. Flickinger JC, Kondziolka D, Lunsford LD, et al. A multi-institutional analysis of complication outcomes after arteriovenous malformation radiosurgery. Int J Radiat Oncol Biol Phys 1999;44: 67–74.

73. Flickinger JC, Kondziolka D, Maitz AH, et al. An analysis of the dose-response for arteriovenous malformation radiosurgery and other factors affecting obliteration. Radiother Oncol 2002;63: 347–54.

74. Hosobuchi Y, Fabrikant JI, Lyman JT. Stereotactic heavy-particle irradiation of intracranial arteriovenous malformations. Appl Neurophysiol 1987;50: 248–52.

75. Kjellberg RN, Abbe M. Stereotactic Bragg peak proton beam therapy. In: Lunsford LD, editor. Modern stereotactic neurosurgery. 1st edition. Boston: Martinus Nijhoff; 1988. p. 463–70.

76. Loeffler JS, Siddon RL, Wen PY, et al. Stereotactic radiosurgery of the brain using a standard linear accelerator: a study of early and late effects. Radiother Oncol 1990;17:311–21.

77. Marks MP, Delapaz RL, Fabrikant JI, et al. Intracranial vascular malformations: imaging of charged-particle radiosurgery. Part II. Complications. Radiology 1988; 168:457–62.

78. Chen HI, Burnett MG, Huse JT, et al. Recurrent late cerebral necrosis with aggressive characteristics after radiosurgical treatment of an arteriovenous malformation. Case report. J Neurosurg 2006;105: 455–60.

79. Lynn M, Friedman W. Hyperbaric oxygen in the treatment of a radiosurgical complication: technical case report. Neurosurgery 2007;60:E579.

80. Yamamoto M, Ban S, Ide M, et al. Diffuse white matter ischemic lesion appearing 7 years after stereotactic radiosurgery for cerebral arteriovenous malformations: case report. Neurosurgery 1997; 41:1405–9.

81. Yamamoto M, Hara M, Ide M, et al. Radiation-related adverse effects observed on neuro-imaging several years after radiosurgery for cerebral arteriovenous malformations. Surg Neurol 1998;49:385–97.

82. Yamamoto M, Ide M, Jimbo M, et al. Middle cerebral artery stenosis caused by relatively low-dose irradiation with stereotactic radiosurgery for cerebral arteriovenous malformations: case report. Neurosurgery 1997;41:474–7.

83. Yamamoto Y, Coffey RJ, Nichols DA, et al. Interim report on the radiosurgical treatment of cerebral arteriovenous malformations. The influence of size, dose, time, and technical factors on obliteration rate. J Neurosurg 1995;83: 832–7.

84. Kihlstrom L, Guo WY, Karlsson B, et al. Magnetic resonance imaging of obliterated arteriovenous malformations up to 23 years after radiosurgery. J Neurosurg 1997;86:589–93.

85. Hara M, Nakamura M, Shiokawa Y, et al. Delayed cyst formation after radiosurgery for cerebral arteriovenous malformation: two case reports. Minim Invasive Neurosurg 1998;41:40–5.

86. Karlsson B, Kihlstrom L, Lindquist C, et al. Gamma knife surgery for previously irradiated arteriovenous malformations. Neurosurgery 1998;42:1–5.

87. Karlsson B, Lindqvist M, Blomgren H, et al. Long-term results after fractionated radiation therapy for large brain arteriovenous malformations. Neurosurgery 2005;57:42–9.

88. Maesawa S, Flickinger JC, Kondziolka D, et al. Repeated radiosurgery for incompletely obliterated arteriovenous malformation. J Neurosurg 2000;92: 961–70.

89. Mirza-Aghazadeh J, Andrade-Souza YM, Zadeh G, et al. Radiosurgical retreatment for brain arteriovenous malformation. Can J Neurol Sci 2006;33:189–94.

90. Raza SM, Jabbour S, Thai QA, et al. Repeat stereotactic radiosurgery for high-grade and large intracranial arteriovenous malformations. Surg Neurol 2007;68:24–34.

91. Schlienger M, Nataf F, Lefkopoulos D, et al. Repeat linear accelerator radiosurgery for cerebral arteriovenous malformations. Int J Radiat Oncol Biol Phys 2003;56:529–36.

92. Foote KD, Friedman WA, Ellis TL, et al. Salvage retreatment after failure of radiosurgery in patients with arteriovenous malformations. J Neurosurg 2003;98:337–41.

93. Pollock BE, Kline RW, Stafford SL, et al. The rationale and technique of staged-volume arteriovenous malformation radiosurgery. Int J Radiat Oncol Biol Phys 2000;48:817–24.

94. Sirin S, Kondziolka D, Niranjan A, et al. Prospective staged volume radiosurgery for large arteriovenous malformations: indications and outcomes in otherwise untreatable patients. Neurosurgery 2006;58:17–27.

95. Dawson RC, Tarr RW, Hecht ST, et al. Treatment of arteriovenous malformations of the brain with combined embolization and stereotactic radiosurgery: results after 1 and 2 years. AJNR Am J Neuroradiol 1990;11:857–64.

96. Lemme-Plaghos L, Schonholz C, Willis R. Combination of embolization and radiosurgery in the treatment of arteriovenous malformations. In: Steiner L, editor. Radiosurgery: baseline and trends. New York: Raven Press; 1992. p. 195–208.

97. Mathis JA, Barr JD, Horton JA, et al. The efficacy of particulate embolization combined with stereotactic radiosurgery for treatment of large arteriovenous

malformations of the brain. AJNR Am J Neuroradiol 1995;16:299–306.

98. Guo WY, Wikholm G, Karlsson B, et al. Combined embolization and gamma knife radiosurgery for cerebral arteriovenous malformations. Acta Radiol 1993;34:600–6.

99. Gobin YP, Laurent A, Merienne L, et al. Treatment of brain arteriovenous malformations by embolization and radiosurgery. J Neurosurg 1996;85:19–28.

100. Henkes H, Nahser HC, Berg-Dammer E, et al. Endovascular therapy of brain AVMs prior to radiosurgery. Neurol Res 1998;20:479–92.

101. Zabel-du Bois A, Milker-Zabel S, Huber P, et al. Risk of hemorrhage and obliteration rates of LINAC-based radiosurgery for cerebral arteriovenous malformations treated after prior partial embolization. Int J Radiat Oncol Biol Phys 2007; 68:999–1003.

Stereotactic Radiosurgery of Intracranial Cavernous Malformations

Gábor Nagy, MD, PhD[a], Andras A. Kemeny, FRCS, MD[b,*]

KEYWORDS

- Basal ganglia • Brainstem • Cavernous malformation • Epilepsy • Stereotactic radiosurgery
- Thalamus

KEY POINTS

- The natural history of cerebral cavernous malformations (CMs) is varied, according to their anatomic position. Although many are silent and the risk of persisting disability after 1 bleed is low, some lesions behave more aggressively. At present, it is not possible to predict future behavior at presentation, but subsequent hemorrhages often cause cumulative morbidity, particularly from deep-seated lesions.
- Surgery for symptomatic hemispheric CMs, and a subset of deep-seated eloquent lesions, may be safe if performed by experienced clinicians.
- Stereotactic radiosurgery is a safe and effective treatment alternative for cerebral CM. There is a dramatic decrease in rebleed rate after a 2-year latency period, whereas using current protocols radiation-induced morbidity is low.
- We propose a simple management algorithm that recommends early stereotactic radiosurgery, even after only 1 event in neurologically intact or minimally disabled patients harboring deep-seated CMs.

INTRODUCTION

A recent international survey showed that there is "considerable uncertainty amongst cerebrovascular experts" about the optimal management of cerebral cavernous malformations (CMs).[1] Of the 194 responders (153 of them being neurosurgeons) seeing a median of 5 new patients per year, the management preferences varied depending on location and clinical course, hemorrhagic brainstem CM being the most controversial issue. Consensus seems to exist in the treatment of choice for hemispheric (lobar) CM: microsurgery when symptomatic and observation for incidental lesions. However, considerable differences were found for lesions in the brainstem: for patients with 2 bleeds, 59% of the responders advocated surgery, 14% stereotactic radiosurgery (SRS), 7% conservative management, and 20% were unsure. The management of deep-seated lesions with only 1 or without hemorrhage is even more contentious.

Radiosurgery was introduced as a treatment option for CM based on the assumption that the vessels would respond similarly to true arteriovenous malformations that had been proved to undergo

Funding Sources: None.

Conflicts of Interest: None.

[a] Department of Neuro-Oncology, National Institute of Neurosciences, Amerikai út 57, Budapest 1145, Hungary; [b] National Centre for Stereotactic Radiosurgery, Royal Hallamshire Hospital, Glossop Road, Sheffield, South Yorkshire S10 2JF, UK

* Corresponding author.

E-mail address: aakemeny@gmail.com

thrombo-obliteration after radiosurgery.[2] Since then, increasing worldwide clinical experience together with few documented histopathologic cases seem to support the initial intuition. Therefore, SRS is recommended as a treatment option for cerebral CM with repeated hemorrhages when they are deemed surgically inaccessible.[3] However, skepticism still exists among some experts about its effectiveness and safety. CM are angiographically occult vascular malformations and therefore no reliable radiological measure (end point) is currently available to show their cure by SRS. Thus, the proponents' argument is based on observational patient statistics of heterogenous quality. It is therefore uncertain whether the efficacy allows SRS to be an alternative for surgery. Furthermore, as do all interventions, it also has side effects and a proportion of treated patients become permanently disabled by adverse radiation effects or hemorrhage. The untreated natural history is that of stepwise neurologic deterioration. These factors often lead to a dilemma: where surgery is not offered, is it safe enough to recommend SRS instead of having a wait-and-watch policy for a neurologically intact patient?[4]

Reflecting on this dilemma, we recently analyzed our current Sheffield, United Kingdom, practice, finding SRS to be safe and apparently effective. At the same time, the poor natural history seemed to be supported by the worse status of those who came for treatment only after more than 1 bleed. Therefore, we recommended radiosurgical treatment early, soon after the first presentation.[5] This article summarizes the current knowledge of natural history, surgical treatment, and radiosurgical treatment, focusing mainly on deep eloquent cavernous malformations, which, together with our growing experience and that of others,[6] reinforces our current practice to confidently recommend early radiosurgical intervention.

NATURAL HISTORY OF CAVERNOUS MALFORMATIONS

Cerebral CM (also known as cavernomas, cavernous angiomas, or cavernous hemangiomas) with distinct pathologic and magnetic resonance imaging (MRI) characteristics compose a large proportion of the previously described angiographically occult vascular malformations[7–9] with an estimated prevalence of 0.15% to 0.9%.[10–13] Seventy-six percent of the lesions are located supratentorially, 8% in the basal ganglia/thalamus, and 18% in the brainstem. Multiple CM are found in 19% of patients,[14] more frequently in familiar forms that comprise at least 6% of all cases.[9] Contemporary population-based prospective studies

detected approximately 6 cases/million/y in Scotland, with 47% to 60% of them being asymptomatic.[15,16] Only 9.3% of the lesions initially found incidentally or presented with seizures go on to cause hemorrhage or focal neurologic deficit within 5 years, but the risk of a second event increases to 42.4%.[16] When patients become symptomatic, typically in their 30s, 37% present with seizures, 36% with hemorrhage, 23% with headaches, and 22% with focal neurologic deficits.[14] Deep eloquent cavernous malformations (with an estimated incidence between 1.2 and 3.2 cases/million/y), once they become symptomatic, seem to behave more aggressively.[5,17–19]

What Counts as a Clinical Hemorrhage?

Part of the problem with understanding the natural history of CM is confusion over what constitutes a hemorrhage.[20] Not all clinical events (acute neurologic deterioration) are associated with evidence of concurrent hemorrhage.[21] However, ultrastructural studies suggest a compromised blood-brain barrier at the site of a CM that may lead to a chronic erythrocyte leak into the surrounding brain and consequently to deposition of hemosiderin in perilesional tissue in the absence of clinically significant hemorrhage.[22] The evidence of a hemosiderin ring around the lesion is the sine qua non of a CM regardless of clinical history,[20] but, without a distinction between clinical and radiological hemorrhage, calculating first-ever bleed and rebleed rates is meaningless. However, as discussed later, the first clinical hemorrhage seems to have a major impact on later behavior and therefore this understanding is fundamental in therapeutic decision making. For pragmatic reasons, we therefore advocate accepting the definition described by Al-Shahi Salman and colleagues[23]: a hemorrhage is a clinical event with acute or subacute onset of symptoms with radiological, pathologic, surgical, or cerebrospinal fluid evidence of recent extralesional or intralesional hemorrhage, whereas simply the existence of a hemosiderin ring or the sole increase in diameter are not considered as hemorrhage.

Risk of Hemorrhage and its Morbidity

Retrospective studies estimate first-ever hemorrhage rates between 0.1% and 2.7%/lesion/y[10,24,25] and from 0.25% to 2.7%/person/y[10,24–26] based on the assumption of lesion presence since birth. Despite evidence of de novo CM formation,[27,28] prospective studies gave similar hemorrhage rates: 0.7% to 1.1%/lesion/y[11,27] and 1.6% to 3.1%/person/y.[21,26,29,30] The range for the risk of a first hemorrhage may not only reflect different definitions of hemorrhage, but small and heterogenous patient populations with short observation periods. Distinct proportions of deep-seated CMs may also count, because the annual risk of hemorrhage specifically from brainstem and thalamic/basal ganglia CM has generally been estimated to be higher (2.3%–6.8%/person/y).[18,19] It is not clear whether deep-seated CMs are more prone to bleeding, or whether any bleed is just more likely to be symptomatic because of higher functional density.

A first bleed may destabilize a CM and increase the risk of further bleeding, which is supported by most studies with only a few exceptions.[29,31] Prospective studies described rebleed rate with estimates between 4.5% and 22.9% per year,[26,32] and retrospective studies focusing on deep eloquent lesions found even higher rebleed rates, between 21% and 60% per year,[24,33,34] and the cumulative incidence of rebleed was 56% after 5 years, and 72% after 10 years.[35] Moreover, a recent prospective study found that even lesions that presented with nonhemorrhagic symptoms have higher risk of bleeding than incidental lesions (2.18% and 0.33% per year, respectively).[30] It is debated whether increased rebleed risk is time limited and decreases a few years after the first hemorrhage (temporal clustering)[16,30,34,35] or whether it remains stable for many years after presentation.[5,36] Part of the confusion may again relate to what constitutes the first bleed, but it may also be that there are distinct populations, and that some CMs behave aggressively with a high risk of rebleeding temporarily or for a longer period after a first hemorrhage, whereas other malformations are more quiescent. If this is the case, the proportion of more aggressive lesions is unknown and currently it is not possible to predict from a first bleed which pattern of behavior a CM will follow.

Not only hemorrhage rate, but permanent morbidity and mortality are higher for deep eloquent lesions.[32,37,38] A single bleed leads to persisting neurologic deficit in up to 40% to 60% of patients harboring deep eloquent CMs and also carries substantial risk of mortality,[5,24,32,33] and each subsequent bleeding episode cumulatively increases the chance for permanent disability (**Table 1**).[5,37]

SURGERY FOR DEEP ELOQUENT CAVERNOUS MALFORMATIONS

For symptomatic hemispheric CMs located superficially, surgery is usually safe and effective.[46] For deep-seated lesions surgery is generally recommended if the lesions that reach the pial or

ependymal surface, or are approachable through an accessible noneloquent surgical corridor, bleed repeatedly with progressive neurologic deficits or cause significant mass effect.[19,47] Because the number of candidates for surgery in this subgroup is low, most centers have limited surgical experience, resecting only maximum of a couple of dozen of such lesions over decades. Only few centers treated more than 100 brainstem CMs surgically and even their results are inferior to those of hemispheric resections. The surgical risks derive from the eloquent anatomy, the lack of safe surgical corridors (particularly if hematoma is absent), and the frequently minimal preoperative neurologic deficit, combined with limited specific experience dealing with this disorder. Therefore, there is a general reluctance in operating on patients with no or minimal disability or with no more than 1 hemorrhage from deep-seated lesions. In the large series, persisting surgical morbidity was found in between 11% and 36% with treatment-related mortality between 0% and 4.7%. Moreover, the annual postsurgical bleed risk was between 0.5% and 2%, indicating that even after surgical resection, which is supposed to be the definitive cure, residual or recurrent lesions continue to threaten patients with persisting bleed risk (see **Table 1**).[34,39–41] The rate of recurrence in pediatric patients is even higher.[45] A recent meta-analysis performed on 68 surgical series reporting 1390 patients with brainstem CMs found 14% persisting morbidity and 1.5% mortality. Total resection was achieved in 91%, and 62% of partially resected lesions rebled with 6% mortality.[48] The same group reviewed 103 lesions located to the thalamus and basal ganglia and found similar results: 10% persisting morbidity with 1.9% surgical mortality and 89% resection rate.[19] Thus, although it is an effective salvage treatment, surgery as a prevention is not considered in patients harboring deep-seated CMs with no or minimal neurologic deficit.

RADIOSURGERY FOR CAVERNOUS MALFORMATIONS
Effect of Radiosurgery on Histopathology

The use of SRS for surgically high-risk, angiographically occult vascular malformations was initially based on the assumption that most of these lesions were partially thrombosed arteriovenous malformations and therefore the vessels would respond similarly to true arteriovenous malformations that had been proved to be obliterated by SRS.[49] Later histopathologic studies found CM to be the commonest form of angiographically occult vascular malformation.[8] This happened in

Table 1
Permanent morbidity, related mortality, and estimated rebleed rates in major series reporting different management options for deep cavernous malformations

Investigators	Patients	Permanent Morbidity (%)	Related Mortality (%)	Rebleeds per Patient per Year (%)
Observation				
Fritschi et al,[24] 1994	30	36.7	20	21
Aiba et al,[32] 1995	22	36	4.5	11–21.5[a]
Porter et al,[33] 1999	12	42	8	30[b]
Surgery				
Wang et al,[34] 2003	137	27.7	0.7	0.5
Abla et al,[39] 2011	260[c]	36	2.3	2
Dukatz et al,[40] 2011	71	11	0	N/A[d]
Pandey et al,[41] 2013	176	11.3	4.7	1.5
Radiosurgery				
Kida,[42] 2009	84	N/A	2.4	7.1–1.8[e]
Lunsford et al,[43] 2010	103[f]	ARE, 1	1	10.8–1.06
Nagy et al,[5] 2010	113	ARE, 7.3	0	5.1–1.3
	—	HEM, 7.3	—	15–2.4[g]
Lee et al,[44] 2012	50[h]	ARE, 4.1	0	3.3–1.74

Abbreviations: ARE, adverse radiation effects; HEM, hemorrhage related; N/A, not applicable.
   [a] For basal ganglia being the lower, brainstem the higher rate.
   [b] Estimated retrospectively analyzing 100 cases (both surgical and conservative group).
   [c] Adults only, another 40 pediatric patients from the same group with similar permanent morbidity, but higher recurrence.[45]
   [d] Recurrence rate was 2.8%.
   [e] For radiosurgery, rebleed rate is given within the first 2 years and thereafter separately.
   [f] Ninety-three in deep location.
   [g] Low-risk group (ie, no more than 1 bleed before radiosurgery) in upper line; high-risk group (ie, at least 2 hemorrhages before radiosurgery) in lower line.
   [h] Brainstem only.
   Data from Refs.[5,10,24,32–34,39,40,42–44]

parallel with better definition of the radiological appearance of CM[7,27] and with early clinical experience of radiosurgical treatment, suggesting that these lesions would respond indeed similarly to true arteriovenous malformations.[2]

It is well documented that radiation induces hyalinization and thickening of the wall of the endothelial-lined vascular channels in arteriovenous malformations.[50,51] Similar radiation-induced vasculopathy is observed in CMs resected surgically after radiation. Gewirtz and colleagues[52] reported histologic examination of 8 CMs removed because of recurrent hemorrhages 1 to 10 years after irradiation showing fibrinoid necrosis to be unique to the irradiated lesions, but none of the lesions had completely thrombosed. Karlsson and colleagues[53] showed that 75% of a CM resected 5 years after SRS had been obliterated without change in its size. Nyáry and colleagues[54] performed detailed histologic examination on a thalamic CM removed 1 year after 40 Gy of fractionated irradiation. Comparison with nonirradiated lesions showed endothelial cell destruction, marked fibrosis, with hyaline degeneration and scar tissue formation. In addition, most of the vessels were obliterated, but there were also signs of neovascularization similar to subtotally obliterated arteriovenous malformations. These specimens came from lesions that remained symptomatic after radiation, and those rendered silent by the treatment may show complete response if they are removed for analysis. It is also postulated that scarring thickens the wall even without full obliteration and stabilizes such a low-pressure lesion sufficiently to prevent it from rebleeding.

MRI after SRS fails to show a change in lesion appearance (**Figs. 1** and **2**). Approximately half of the lesions shrank and another half remained similar in size in larger studies,[42,43] and only a few exceptional enlarging lesions have been reported.[42,55,56] Although proportion of true growth is higher in untreated populations,[27,28] on MRI lesions after radiosurgical treatment statistically appear as heterogenous as those without

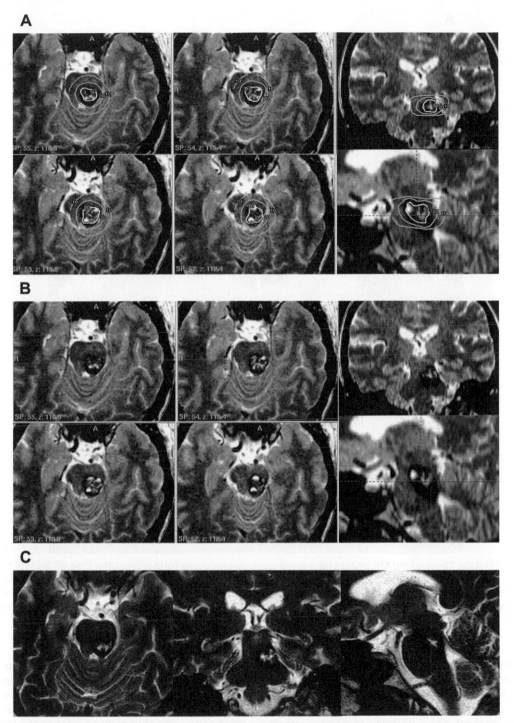

Fig. 1. (*A*) Treatment planning using T2-weighted MR images for an upper pons cavernous malformation of type II appearance[27] typical of lesions treated with radiosurgery. (*Red line*, lesion marked by neuroradiologist within the hemosiderin ring. *Yellow line*, 50% isodose line. *Green lines*, 20% and 10% isodose lines.) (*B*) T2-weighted MR images of the same lesion at treatment without treatment planning lines, and (*C*) 2 years after radiosurgical treatment; despite lacking further hemorrhages, no significant change in size or appearance is visible.

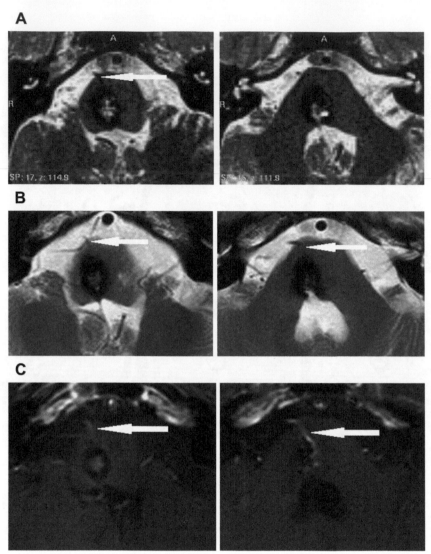

Fig. 2. (*A*) Axial T2-weighted MR images for a lower pons cavernous malformation at the time of, and (*B*) 6 years after, radiosurgical treatment. As in **Fig. 1**, no significant change in size or appearance is visible despite lacking further hemorrhages. (*C*) Axial T1-weighted postgadolinium follow-up MR images of the same lesion 6 years after treatment. Intact developmental venous anomaly is visible both on T2-weighted and on T1-weighted postgadolinium MR images in association with the treated cavernous malformation (*white arrows*).

treatment. More importantly, using current imaging techniques it is impossible to show the cure of an individual CM and to tell whether it is secured from a further bleed. Therefore we only recommend imaging when clinically significant events occur, and then to distinguish between radiation-induced edema,[2,56] bleed, or event without radiological change.[5]

Effect of Radiosurgery on Hemorrhage Rate

The difficulties in interpreting these events, particularly when attempts are made to account for pre-diagnosis clinical events, are mentioned earlier. The primary aim of SRS is to reduce the risk of future bleeding. This aim is reported by most radiosurgical studies comparing pretreatment and posttreatment bleed rates after a latency of 2 to 3 years (**Table 2**). The first report of large clinical series with sufficient follow-up time was published in 1995 by Kondziolka and colleagues.[2] Rebleeding rate decreased from 32% per patient-year before treatment to 8.8% within the first 2 years after treatment and to 1.1% thereafter. Recent updates on these data, including more patients and longer follow-up, confirmed the initial results (32.5% before treatment, and 10.8% and 1.06% posttreatment rebleed rates within and after 2 years).[43] Ninety percent of the lesions in this study were located in deep eloquent regions, and analyzing the cohort of only brainstem cases gave similar results.[62] Other contemporary radiosurgical series focusing on deep eloquent lesions,[5,44,58,63] and studies analyzing mixed populations of lobar and deep cavernous malformations,[60] confirmed this finding (see **Tables 1** and **2**). However, this is not a universal finding, which may reflect patient selection and varied interpretation of what counts as a hemorrhagic event. Amin-Hanjani and colleagues[57] analyzed 95 patients treated by proton beam therapy between 1977 and 1993. There was a reduction in annual rebleed rate to 4.5% from a pretreatment 17.4% only after a 2-year period of temporary increase (22.4%), and Karlsson and colleagues[53] found that bleed rate remained high and decreased only 4 years after treating 22 patients with SRS.

Although most of the published literature suggests that the reduction in rebleed rate of CMs with multiple hemorrhages after a 2-year latency period is caused by the radiobiological effect of the treatment, this has been questioned. The argument is that hemorrhages may occur in clusters, and thus the apparent decrease in bleed rate is the natural history of the condition rather than an effect of radiosurgery.[4,35] This possibility seems unlikely, because the evidence for hemorrhage clustering has been challenged by the finding that those lesions with long pretreatment history of repeated hemorrhages seem to maintain a high rate of events for many years.[5,36] Also, the time course of the observed reduction in rebleed rates after SRS parallels the time course of histologic changes known to develop after irradiation.

Morbidity After Radiosurgery

Morbidity and its severity in untreated cases are both significantly associated with hemorrhage, exacerbated by repeated hemorrhage, and are seen more readily when CMs are in deep eloquent locations. Because the beneficial effect of SRS is expected only after a latency period and the risk of hemorrhage never seems to reach zero, morbidity caused by posttreatment hemorrhage should also be counted. We found that 7.3% of the patients had persisting neurologic deterioration caused by posttreatment hemorrhages. After a bleed, the likelihood of permanent deficit was the same with posttreatment hemorrhages as with pretreatment hemorrhages, suggesting that the benefit of SRS is not to reduce the severity but the frequency of bleeds.[5]

Early studies reported higher radiation-associated persisting complication rates (adverse radiation effects) reflecting poor delineation with computed tomography (CT) or less conformal MRI localization and higher dose protocols.[53,57,58] We treated 7 patients with deep eloquent CMs between 1987 and 1990 using CT planning and prescription doses between 15 and 20 Gy, and the rate of adverse radiation effects was unacceptably high.[65] Therefore, it was not until 1995 that we restarted radiosurgical treatment of these lesions with more conformal MRI-based planning and lower prescription doses (typically 12–15 Gy).[5] Our contemporary treatment protocol includes highly conformal treatment planning (the malformation is defined strictly within the hemosiderin ring [see **Fig. 1**], and associated developmental venous anomalies are preserved [see **Fig. 2**]) and prescription dose less than 20 Gy.[6] Such recent studies have reported low complication rates (1%–7.3%) resulting in only mild persisting morbidity, and mortality related to the treated lesion was negligible (see **Table 2**). Between 1995 and 2012, we treated 314 lesions in 285 patients. Of these, 191 lesions in 186 patients were located in deep eloquent regions. Reflecting our aim to move toward earlier active treatment and, in parallel to the increasing worldwide experience on the safety and effectiveness of treating deep eloquent CMs, our treatment numbers increased from an annual 3 to 4 patients before 2000 to an average of 12 patients between 2001 and 2011, and to 26 treatments last year. When publishing our current practice in 2010, we treated 46% of the symptomatic deep CMs presenting in our catchment area with SRS and estimated to treat 10% to 30% of newly diagnosed deep-seated CMs in the United Kingdom. We concluded that the geographic difference represented a reluctance to refer these lesions for SRS, owing to the perceived conflicting evidence on the safety and effectiveness of SRS.[5] Because the number of treated lesions almost doubled in 2012 (43% of the estimated newly diagnosed lesions in the country), we think that the argument for early radiosurgical treatment is winning.

The Effect of Radiosurgery on Epilepsy Related to Cavernous Malformations

For patients with intractable epilepsy, surgical resection of hemispheric CM is the treatment of choice because it is associated with low morbidity and high effectiveness.[46] However, several conditions may warrant treatment alternatives, including eloquently located lesions, the patient's medical condition, or the patient's preference.

Table 2
Summary of major radiosurgical series

Authors	Patients (lesions) (n)	Deep (n)	Superficial (n)	Pre-trt 1st bleed (/year)	Pre-trt rebleed (/year)	Post-trt bleed (/year)	Post-trt bleed until 2yr (/year)	Post-trt bleed after 2yr (/year)	Permanent ARE (%)	Post-trt bleed related morbidity (%)	Related mortality (%)	Comments
Amin-Hanjani et al,[57] 1998	95 (98)	74	24	N/A	16.9	9.3	22.4	4.5	30.5	21	8.4	1. Proton beam 2. 1977–1993 3. CT or MRI plan
Chang et al,[64] 1998	57	52	5	N/A	N/A	N/A	12.3	1.9	11	N/A	3.5	1. Helium or LINAC 2. 1983–1994
Karlsson et al,[53] 1998	22	13	9	N/A	N/A	8	10	N/A	22	N/A	0	1. Gamma knife 2. 1985–1996 3. CT or MRI plan
Pollock et al,[58] 2000	17	17	0	N/A	24.8	N/A	8.8	2.9	41	N/A	0	1. Gamma knife 2. 1990–1997 3. MRI plan
Kida & Hasegawa,[59] 2004	152	87	65	N/A	31.8[a]	3.2	8[b]	<5	N/A	N/A	2	1. Gamma knife 2. 1991–2001
Liu et al,[60] 2005	125	63	49	N/A	29.2	6.5	10.3	3.3	3.2	9.6	0	1. Gamma knife 2. 1993–2002
Liscák et al,[56] 2005	112	50	62	N/A	N/A	N/A	N/A	N/A[c]	4.5	N/A	1.8	1. Gamma knife 2. 1993–2000 3. CT or MRI plan

Study												Gamma knife
Kida,[42] 2009	84	84	0	N/A	N/A	4.2	7.1	1.8	N/A	N/A	2.4	1. Gamma knife 2. 1995–2005 3. CT or MRI plan
Wang et al,[61] 2010	96	13	83	N/A	N/A	0.9	4.2	<2.1	5.2	N/A	0	1. Gamma knife 2. 1988–2005 3. CT or MRI plan
Lunsford et al,[43] 2010[d]	103	93	10	N/A	32.5	4.46	10.8	1.06	1	N/A	1	1. Gamma knife 2. 1988–2005 3. CT or MRI plan
Monaco et al,[62] 2010	68[e]	68	0	N/A	32.38	N/A	8.2	1.37	1.5	N/A	2.9	1. Gamma knife 2. 1988–2005 3. CT or MRI plan
Nagy et al,[5] 2010[f]	113 (118)	118	0	2.29[g] / 2.9	30.5	N/A / N/A	5.1 / 15	1.3 / 2.4	7.3	7.3	0	1. Gamma knife 2. 1995–2008 3. MRI plan
Park & Hwang,[63] 2012	20	20	0	N/A	39.5	N/A	8.2	0	5	0	0	1. Gamma knife 2. 2005–2010 3. MRI plan
Lee et al,[44] 2012	49 (50)[h]	50	0	N/A	31.3	N/A	3.3	1.74	4.1	N/A	0	1. Gamma knife 2. 1993–2010 3. MRI plan

Abbreviations: CT, computed tomography; LINAC, linear accelerator.

[a] During 5 years prior to radiosurgery.
[b] First year after treatment.
[c] Definition and calculation of bleed is not suitable for comparison to others.
[d] Latest report from this group (earlier reports not indicated in the table separately).
[e] Brainstem only.
[f] Only current treatment technique, first report with older cases not indicated in the table.
[g] First line "low risk", second line "high risk" group.
[h] Brainstem only, earlier report from the same group includes all cases.[59]

A retrospective multicenter study on gamma knife treatment in 49 patients with long lasting (7.5 years) epilepsy refractory to medical therapy showed that 53% of the patients were seizure free (Engel class IA and B) within a mean of 4 months after treatment, 20% showed highly significant improvement (class II), and 26% little or no improvement (class III and IV).[66] Patients with CMs located in the mesial temporal lobe did worse than those treated in other locations. More recent studies found similar results: 39% to 54% of the patients became seizure free (class I), and 14% to 20.5% improved significantly (class II).[60,61] Ninety percent of the patients with short history of epilepsy (≤3 years) improved, whereas only 38.5% with longer lasting epileptic disease improved.[61] Persisting side effects were negligible in all studies. A recent single-center study compared surgical and radiosurgical treatment and found no significant difference between the outcomes of the two groups, although the surgical group tended to do better and analysis of a larger cohort might have given significant difference (86.7% class I, 13.3% class II vs 64.3% class I and 28.6% class II in the surgical and radiosurgical groups, respectively).[67] Thus, SRS seems to be an effective treatment alternative for CM causing epilepsy.

Perspectives on Radiosurgery in the Management of Cavernous Malformations

The lack of quality evidence makes it impossible to propose a universal guideline for the management of cerebral CM.[68] In our view, all 3 treatment modalities (conservative, surgical, and radiosurgical) should play an important role in the management of patients with CM. The indications for each approach, although overlapping, are complementary and not competitive. For this reason, direct comparisons of outcomes after the resection or SRS of CM are misleading,[57] which also questions the scope of future randomized controlled trials, because the cohort in which equipoise exists between the two modalities will be small. Future attempts should focus on refining the definition of the limitations and indications of each modality; this is particularly true for SRS, because increasing positive experience with current radiosurgical protocols moves SRS from a niche treatment of inaccessible lesions with multiple bleeds toward a more confident use early after their presentation as a preventive treatment.

Based on available data reviewed earlier, we propose a treatment algorithm (Fig. 3). Incidental hemispheric CMs located superficially can be observed because the chance for becoming symptomatic is low, whereas, unless patient factors preclude it, surgical removal of symptomatic hemispheric lesions is the treatment of choice. In such cases, SRS can be reserved as an alternative option, for eloquent cortical position or dictated by patient choice. Deep-seated lesions seem to be more challenging because of their unpredictable nature and higher morbidity regardless of treatment modality. For an incidental deep-seated lesion, both observation and SRS seem to be valid

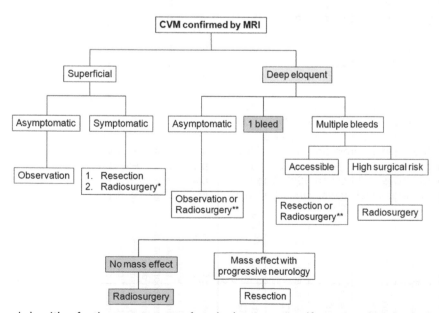

Fig. 3. Proposed algorithm for the management of cerebral cavernous malformations (CVM). *Surgery is first option in most cases, but radiosurgery is a valid alternative. **Both modalities appear to be effective, but currently there is no evidence to demonstrate superiority of either.

options. In this situation, the low rate of radiation-induced morbidity after SRS may be outweighed by the potential future benefits. For lesions that present with a bleed but do not cause mass effect or progressive neurologic deterioration, early radiosurgical treatment 3 to 6 months after the first bleed (allowing for clinical recovery and resolution of hematoma) is recommended because the consequences of potential subsequent bleeds seem to be more severe than radiation-induced side effects. For lesions with multiple bleeds, management is primarily defined by surgical accessibility, because these lesions have already been proved to behave more aggressively, therefore even a higher risk surgical resection offering an instant and likely definitive protection from further hemorrhages is at times accepted. Radiosurgery for those patients who carry unacceptable surgical risk remains an alternative even in this group. However, we agree with a recent guideline that the final treatment decision for an individual patient is also influenced by the neurosurgeon's experience and by patient preference.[6]

By reviewing the current radiosurgical literature, we found heterogenous reports with distinct measures of natural history, posttreatment bleed rates, and morbidity (see **Table 2**). Therefore, we propose standardized reporting criteria for the radiosurgical community for improved data collection, because this seems to be the most realistic way to get a better view on the safety and effectiveness of the technique in the near future (**Table 3**).

1. Al-Shahi Salman and colleagues[23] published a thorough list of clinical variables to be reported in CM research. Based on this recommendation, we propose to collect and report a minimum of the following patient and lesion characteristics before treatment: age at presentation and treatment, sex, mode of clinical presentation and presenting symptoms, family history, multiplicity, location, size, and associated venous anomalies. Retrospective annual first-bleed rate for treated lesions (per lesion per year) should be reported separately from annual rebleed rate until treatment (if the latter is applicable). For a treated lesion population, the annual rate of first-ever bleed is calculated with the assumption of lesion presence since birth as the sum of first hemorrhages divided by the sum of ages at first bleed or at lesion

Table 3
Proposal for reporting standards for radiosurgery of cavernous malformations

Standards	Comments
Patient and lesion characteristics before treatment	
Age at presentation and treatment	
Sex, family history	
Presenting symptoms	
Persisting deficits	Modified Rankin Score
Multiplicity	
Rate of first bleed and rebleed	Per treated lesion per year
Bleeds 0, 1, or $\geq$2	
Location: superficial/deep seated	To be analyzed separately
Nonhemorrhagic clinical events	To be recorded separately
Treatment parameters	Because of its high conformity, gamma knife is considered to be the gold standard for radiosurgical treatment of cavernous malformations
Gross target volume	
Prescription isodose volume	
Prescription dose	
Volumes receiving 10 and 12 Gy	
Paddick Conformity Index	
Gradient Index	
Posttreatment hemorrhage rates	Per treated lesion per year
$\leq$2 y	
>2 y after treatment	
Morbidity related to posttreatment hemorrhages	As reduction in modified Rankin Score
Morbidity related to radiation (ARE)	
Temporary	Duration, requirement for medication
Persisting	As reduction in modified Rankin Score
Radiology	If applicable

detection in case of nonhemorrhagic presentation.[5] Annual rebleed rate is calculated with the use of the time of first bleed as zero for pretreatment observation of the lesion, dividing the number of subsequent bleeds by pretreatment observation years between first hemorrhage and treatment.[2] We recommend analyzing superficial and deep-seated lesions and lesions with zero, 1, or multiple bleeds separately. Treating incidental lesions seems to be not a widely accepted practice, so some may choose to pool them with lesions with single hemorrhage. We recommend accepting the definition of a bleed proposed by Al-Shahi Salman and colleagues,[23] and record nonhemorrhagic clinical events separately.

2. Based on the experience accumulated worldwide over recent decades, gamma knife SRS with current treatment protocol seems to be the most precise radiosurgical treatment of cerebral CM. Therefore, it is our recommendation to treat these lesions with gamma knife SRS and report standardized treatment parameters. The Leksell Gamma Knife Society is in the process of publishing agreed reporting standards for radiosurgery. For this disorder, the following would be a minimum dataset: gross target volume, prescription isodose volume, prescription dose, volumes receiving 10 and 12 Gy, Paddick Conformity Index, and Gradient Index.

3. Hemorrhage rates should be calculated separately within 2 years after treatment and thereafter. A distinction between hemorrhagic and nonhemorrhagic clinical events and their separate documentation is also recommended.

4. Most papers, to our surprise and disappointment, do not report morbidity related to posttreatment hemorrhages (see **Table 2**). Because a delayed protection is specific to this treatment modality, we think it is fair to record it accurately.

5. Temporary neurologic deficit associated with radiological evidence of perilesional edema, typically presented within 12 months after treatment, are recorded separately. Although not proved for all cases, we recommend recording all persisting neurologic deterioration not related to posttreatment hemorrhage as persisting adverse radiation effect.[5]

6. Because there is currently no radiological measure to predict effectiveness of radiosurgical treatment, in our view routine radiological follow-up is not necessary in the everyday clinical practice.[5] Further research is needed to find an objective radiological measure for cure.

Because several hundred patients have already been treated worldwide in major radiosurgical centers, a meta-analysis of published material using these criteria would be welcome. It would also provide the basis for a future prospective international radiosurgical data collection.

The weakest point of all the available radiosurgical articles is the lack of a control group.[68] Critics of this method advocate a prospective randomized controlled trial to clarify the conflicting issues surrounding SRS.[4,69] Such a trial has already been designed to compare resection and radiosurgery for high-risk CM and included 8 large neurovascular centers in the United States and Canada.[70] However, it was terminated after 1 year because not a single patient had entered into the study.[71] Our experience also suggests that there is difficulty with patient recruitment because most of them wish to decide for themselves the mode of treatment, particularly when the risk of interventions is considered critical. Moreover, there is no consensus about the design of such a trial. As discussed earlier, we consider surgical resection and SRS to be complementary rather than conflicting, so our proposal is for a trial to compare conservative and radiosurgical management early after initial presentation. Prospective international data collection including all detected cases regardless of treatment modality seems to be a more realistic goal, and would act as preparation for a case-control study. Nevertheless, quality evidence from either a prospective randomized trial or a case-control study is needed.

SUMMARY

Stereotactic radiosurgery in the management of cerebral CM remains controversial, although dissenting voices are increasingly in the minority. There is now sufficient evidence supporting the use of SRS for CMs located in the brainstem, thalamus, basal ganglia, or internal capsule, once they become symptomatic. Furthermore, because of the cumulative morbidity of repeated hemorrhages and the low risk of radiation-induced adverse effects, we advocate an early intervention. In our opinion, waiting for the cumulative morbidity of the natural history to justify intervention does not serve the patient well. Carefully designed randomized controlled trials, if their recruitment is successful, might provide even stronger arguments to use SRS in the future. Until then, the radiosurgical community is tasked to provide high-quality data by standardized reporting of their outcomes for this condition.

REFERENCES

1. Al-Shahi Salman R, Chilton L, Mendelow AD, et al. Current treatment practice for cavernous

malformations: international survey [abstract T5-05]. In: proceedings of the 154th Meeting of the Society of British Neurological Surgeons: Dublin, Ireland, October 2009. Br J Neurosurg 2009;23:468–90.

2. Kondziolka D, Lunsford LD, Flickinger JC, et al. Reduction of hemorrhage risk after stereotactic radiosurgery for cavernous malformations. J Neurosurg 1995;83:825–31.

3. Brown RD Jr, Flemming KD, Meyer FB, et al. Natural history, evaluation, and management of intracranial vascular malformations. Mayo Clin Proc 2005; 80:269–81.

4. Steiner L, Karlsson B, Yen CP, et al. Radiosurgery in cavernous malformations: anatomy of a controversy. J Neurosurg 2010;113:16–21.

5. Nagy G, Razak A, Rowe JG, et al. Stereotactic radiosurgery for deep-seated cavernous malformations: a move toward more active, early intervention. J Neurosurg 2010;113:691–9.

6. Niranjan A, Lunsford LD. Stereotactic radiosurgery guidelines for the management of patients with intracranial cavernous malformations. Prog Neurol Surg 2013;27:166–75.

7. Rigamonti D, Drayer BP, Johnson PC, et al. The MRI appearance of cavernous malformations (angiomas). J Neurosurg 1987;67:518–24.

8. Tomlinson FH, Houser OW, Scheithauer BW, et al. Angiographically occult vascular malformations: a correlative study of features on magnetic resonance imaging and histological examination. Neurosurgery 1994;34:792–800.

9. Batra S, Lin D, Recinos PF, et al. Cavernous malformations: natural history, diagnosis and treatment. Nat Rev Neurol 2009;5:659–70.

10. Del Curling O Jr, Kelly DL Jr, Elster AD, et al. An analysis of the natural history of cavernous angiomas. J Neurosurg 1991;75:702–8.

11. Robinson JR, Awad IA, Little JR. Natural history of the cavernous angioma. J Neurosurg 1991;75:709–14.

12. Sage MR, Brophy BP, Sweeney C, et al. Cavernous haemangiomas (angiomas) of the brain: clinically significant lesions. Australas Radiol 1993;37:147–55.

13. Al-Shahi Salman R, Whiteley WN, Warlow C. Screening using whole-body magnetic resonance imaging scanning: who wants an incidentaloma? J Med Screen 2007;14:2–4.

14. Gross BA, Lin N, Du R, et al. The natural history of intracranial cavernous malformations. Neurosurg Focus 2011;30:E24.

15. Al-Shahi R, Bhattacharya JJ, Currie DG, et al. Prospective, population-based detection of intracranial vascular malformations in adults. The Scottish Intracranial Vascular Malformation Study (SIVMS). Stroke 2003;34:1163–9.

16. Al-Shahi Salman R, Hall JM, Horne MA, et al. Untreated clinical course of cerebral cavernous

malformations: a prospective, population-based cohort study. Lancet Neurol 2012;11:217–24.

17. Mathiesen T, Edner G, Kihlström L. Deep and brainstem cavernomas: a consecutive 8-year series. J Neurosurg 2003;99:31–7.

18. Gross BA, Batjer HH, Awad IA, et al. Brainstem cavernous malformations. Neurosurgery 2009;64: E805–18.

19. Gross BA, Batjer HH, Awad IA, et al. Cavernous malformations of the basal ganglia and thalamus. Neurosurgery 2009;65:7–18.

20. Maraire JN, Awad IA. Intracranial cavernous malformations: lesion behavior and management strategies. Neurosurgery 1995;37:591–605.

21. Porter PJ, Willinsky RA, Harper W, et al. Cerebral cavernous malformations: natural history and prognosis after clinical deterioration with or without hemorrhage. J Neurosurg 1997;87:190–7.

22. Clatterbuck R, Eberhart C, Crain B, et al. Ultrastructural and immunocytochemical evidence that an incompetent blood-brain barrier is related to the pathophysiology of cavernous malformations. J Neurol Neurosurg Psychiatry 2001;71:188–92.

23. Al-Shahi Salman R, Berg MJ, Morrison L, et al. Hemorrhage from cavernous malformations of the brain: definition and reporting standards. Stroke 2008;39:3222–30.

24. Fritschi JA, Reulen HJ, Spetzler RF, et al. Cavernous malformations of the brain stem: a review of 139 cases. Acta Neurochir 1994;130:35–46.

25. Kim DS, Park YG, Choi JU, et al. An analysis of the natural history of cavernous malformations. Surg Neurol 1997;48:9–17.

26. Kondziolka D, Lunsford LD, Kestle JR. The natural history of cerebral cavernous malformations. J Neurosurg 1995;83:820–4.

27. Zabramski JM, Wascher TM, Spetzler RF, et al. The natural history of familial cavernous malformations: results of an ongoing study. J Neurosurg 1994;80: 422–32.

28. Pozzati E, Acciarri N, Tognetti F, et al. Growth, subsequent bleeding, and de novo appearance of cerebral cavernous angiomas. Neurosurgery 1996;38:662–70.

29. Moriarity JL, Wetzel M, Clatterbuck RE, et al. The natural history of cavernous malformations: a prospective study of 68 patients. Neurosurgery 1999; 44:1166–71.

30. Flemming KD, Link MJ, Christianson TJ, et al. Prospective hemorrhage risk of intracerebral cavernous malformations. Neurology 2012;78:632–6.

31. Kupersmith MJ, Kalish H, Epstein F, et al. Natural history of brainstem cavernous malformations. Neurosurgery 2001;48:47–53.

32. Aiba T, Tanaka R, Koike T, et al. Natural history of intracranial cavernous malformations. J Neurosurg 1995;83:56–9.

33. Porter RW, Detwiler PW, Spetzler RF, et al. Cavernous malformation of the brain stem: experience with 100 patients. J Neurosurg 1999;90:50–8.

34. Wang CC, Liu A, Zhang JT, et al. Surgical management of brain-stem cavernous malformations: report of 137 cases. Surg Neurol 2003;59:444–54.

35. Barker FG II, Amin-Hanjani S, Butler WE, et al. Temporal clustering of hemorrhages from untreated cavernous malformations of the central nervous system. Neurosurgery 2001;49:15–25.

36. Hasegawa T, McInerney J, Kondziolka D, et al. Long-term results after stereotactic radiosurgery for patients with cavernous malformations. Neurosurgery 2002;50:1190–8.

37. Tung H, Giannotta SL, Chandrasoma PT, et al. Recurrent intraparenchymal hemorrhages from angiographically occult vascular malformations. J Neurosurg 1990;73:174–80.

38. Robinson JR, Awad IA, Magdinec M, et al. Factors predisposing to clinical disability in patients with cavernous malformations of the brain. Neurosurgery 1993;32:730–6.

39. Abla AA, Lekovic GP, Turner JD, et al. Advances in the treatment and outcome of brainstem cavernous malformation surgery: a single-center case series of 300 surgically treated patients. Neurosurgery 2011;68:403–15.

40. Dukatz T, Sarnthein J, Sitter H, et al. Quality of life after brainstem cavernoma surgery in 71 patients. Neurosurgery 2011;69:689–95.

41. Pandey P, Westbroek EM, Gooderham PA, et al. Cavernous malformation of brainstem, thalamus and basal ganglia–a series of 176 patients. Neurosurgery 2013;72(4):573–89.

42. Kida Y. Radiosurgery for cavernous malformations in basal ganglia, thalamus and brainstem. Prog Neurol Surg 2009;22:31–7.

43. Lunsford LD, Khan AA, Niranjan A, et al. Stereotactic radiosurgery for symptomatic solitary cerebral cavernous malformations considered high risk for resection. J Neurosurg 2010;113:23–9.

44. Lee CC, Pan DH, Chung WY, et al. Brainstem cavernous malformations: the role of gamma knife surgery. J Neurosurg 2012;117(Suppl):164–9.

45. Abla AA, Lekovic GP, Garrett M, et al. Cavernous malformations of the brainstem presenting in childhood: surgical experience in 40 patients. Neurosurgery 2010;67:1589–99.

46. Vives KP, Gunel M, Awad IA. Surgical management of supratentorial cavernous malformations. In: Winn HR, editor. Youmans neurological surgery. 5th edition. Philadelphia: WB Saunders; 2003. p. 2305–20.

47. Porter RW, Detwiler PW, Spetzler RF. Surgical technique for resection of cavernous malformations of the brain stem. Operat Tech Neurosurg 2000;3: 124–30.

48. Gross BA, Batjer HH, Awad IA, et al. Brainstem cavernous malformations: 1390 surgical cases from the literature. World Neurosurg 2012. http://dx.doi.org/10.1016/j.wneu.2012.04.002.

49. Kondziolka D, Lunsford LD, Coffey RJ, et al. Stereotactic radiosurgery of angiographically occult vascular malformations: indications and preliminary experience. Neurosurgery 1990;27:892–900.

50. Schneider BF, Eberhard DA, Steiner LE. Histopathology of arteriovenous malformations after gamma knife radiosurgery. J Neurosurg 1997;87: 352–7.

51. Szeifert GT, Timperley WR, Forster DM, et al. Histopathological changes in cerebral arteriovenous malformations following gamma knife radiosurgery. Prog Neurol Surg 2007;20:212–9.

52. Gewirtz RJ, Steinberg GK, Crowly R, et al. Pathological changes in surgically resected angiographically occult vascular malformations after radiation. Neurosurgery 1998;42:738–43.

53. Karlsson B, Kihlström L, Lindquist C, et al. Radiosurgery for cavernous malformations. J Neurosurg 1998;88:293–7.

54. Nyáry I, Major O, Hanzély Z, et al. Histopathological findings in a surgically resected thalamic cavernous hemangioma 1 year after 40-Gy irradiation. J Neurosurg 2005;102(Suppl):56–8.

55. Kim MS, Pyo SY, Jeong YG, et al. Gamma knife surgery for intracranial cavernous hemangioma. J Neurosurg 2005;102(Suppl):102–6.

56. Liscák R, Vladyka V, Simonová G, et al. Gamma knife surgery of brain cavernous hemangiomas. J Neurosurg 2005;102(Suppl):207–13.

57. Amin-Hanjani S, Ogilvy CS, Candia GJ, et al. Stereotactic radiosurgery for cavernous malformations: Kjellberg's experience with proton beam therapy in 98 cases at the Harvard Cyclotron. Neurosurgery 1998;42:1229–36.

58. Pollock BE, Garces YI, Stafford SL, et al. Stereotactic radiosurgery for cavernous malformations. J Neurosurg 2000;93:987–91.

59. Kida Y, Hasegawa T. Radiosurgery for cavernous malformations: results of long-term follow-up. In: Kondziolka D, editor. Radiosurgery, vol. 5. Basel (Switzerland): Karger; 2004. p. 153–60.

60. Liu KD, Chung WY, Wu HM, et al. Gamma knife surgery for cavernous hemangiomas: an analysis of 125 patients. J Neurosurg 2005;102(Suppl):81–6.

61. Wang P, Zhang F, Zhang H, et al. Gamma knife radiosurgery for intracranial cavernous malformations. Clin Neurol Neurosurg 2010;112:474–7.

62. Monaco EA III, Khan AA, Niranjan A, et al. Stereotactic radiosurgery for the treatment of symptomatic brainstem cavernous malformations. Neurosurg Focus 2010;29:E11.

63. Park SH, Hwang SK. Gamma knife radiosurgery for symptomatic brainstem intra-axial cavernous

malformations. World Neurosurg 2012. http://dx.doi.org/10.1016/j.wneu.2012.09.013.

64. Chang SD, Levy RP, Adler JR, et al. Stereotactic radiosurgery of angiographically occult vascular malformations: 14-years experience. Neurosurgery 1998;43:213–21.

65. Mitchell P, Hodgson TJ, Seaman S, et al. Stereotactic radiosurgery and the risk of haemorrhage from cavernous malformations. Br J Neurosurg 2000; 14:96–100.

66. Régis J, Bartolomei F, Kida Y, et al. Radiosurgery for epilepsy associated with cavernous malformation: retrospective study in 49 patients. Neurosurgery 2000;47:1091–7.

67. Hsu PW, Chang CN, Tseng CK, et al. Treatment of epileptogenic cavernomas: surgery versus radiosurgery. Cerebrovasc Dis 2007;24: 116–20.

68. Samarasekera N, Poorthuis M, Kontoh K, et al. Guidelines for the management of cerebral cavernous malformations in adults 2012. Available at: http://www.cavernoma.org.uk/opus473/final_CCM_guidelines_2.pdf. Accessed February 18, 2013.

69. Sheehan J, Schlesinger D. Editorial. Radiosurgery and cavernous malformations. J Neurosurg 2010; 113:689–90.

70. Kondziolka D, Lunsford LD, Flickinger JC. Stereotactic radiosurgery for cavernous malformations. Prog Neurol Surg 1998;14:78–88.

71. Kondziolka D, Lunsford LD. Response to editorial. J Neurosurg 2010;113:21–2.

Stereotactic Radiosurgery of Intracranial Dural Arteriovenous Fistulas

Chun-Po Yen, MD[a], Giuseppe Lanzino, MD[b],
Jason P. Sheehan, MD, PhD[a],*

KEYWORDS

- Arteriovenous fistula • Dura • Stereotactic radiosurgery

KEY POINTS

- Stereotactic radiosurgery resection, and embolization play a role in the treatment of intracranial dural arteriovenous fistulas (dAVF).
- Radiosurgical obliteration of dAVF typically generally requires 1 to 3 years, although symptomatic improvement may precede complete obliteration.
- Stereotactic radiosurgery plays a substantial role in treating dAVF involving a large dural sinus, such as the transverse/sigmoid, the superior sagittal sinus, and indirect cavernous-carotid fistulas.
- Some patients require a combination of treatment approaches.
- The optimal radiosurgical dose for dAVF obliteration seems comparable to that used for intracranial arteriovenous malformations (18–25 Gy).

INTRODUCTION

Dural arteriovenous fistulas (dAVF) represent approximately 15% of all intracranial vascular malformations. Significant gaps remain in the understanding regarding dAVF pathogenesis and treatment. The underlying pathophysiology for the development of intracranial dAVF has been refined with the advancement of several theories, including changes in blood flow dynamics at the site of a pre-existing dural venous thrombosis and increased expression of angiogenic factors, such as vascular-endothelial growth factor (VEGF) in adjacent dural leaflets.[1–3] However, the lack of venous thrombosis in some dAVF can be used to argue against the need for vascular stasis, whereas the absence of clear causative information regarding increases in local VEGF levels in dural samples casts doubt on the importance of these signaling pathways in the creation of dAVF.[4,5]

With the recent advances in endovascular and radiosurgical techniques, along with a better understanding of the pathophysiology and clinical course of intracranial dAVF, individualized treatment that is both effective and safe can be offered to most patients with intracranial dAVF. The choice of the best therapeutic strategy should take into account the clinical presentation, location of the dAVF, angioarchitecture, and patient's preference. Treatment is indicated in patients with disabling symptoms, presence of retrograde cortical venous drainage (CVD), and those with aggressive clinical presentation (hemorrhage or symptoms and signs related to venous hypertension).

Patients with minimal or no symptoms and no evidence of retrograde CVD may be well served

Disclosures: The authors have nothing to disclose.
[a] Department of Neurological Surgery, University of Virginia, PO Box 800212, Charlottesville, VA 22908, USA;
[b] Department of Neurologic Surgery, Mayo Clinic, 200 1st St SW, Rochester, MN 55905, USA
* Corresponding author.
E-mail address: jps2f@virginia.edu

Neurosurg Clin N Am 24 (2013) 591–596
http://dx.doi.org/10.1016/j.nec.2013.05.008
1042-3680/13/$ – see front matter © 2013 Elsevier Inc. All rights reserved.

with observation alone. In these patients, the dAVF are usually located at the transverse/sigmoid junction and the cavernous sinus. In patients with transverse/sigmoid sinus dAVF and no CVD, the natural history is very benign and such cases have a very low risk of hemorrhage.[6] These patients usually present with symptoms related to the high-flow, low-pressure shunt, such as a bruit or localized pain. Alternately, such patients can be completely asymptomatic. In patients with a bruit, the bruit resolves or improves without treatment in approximately 50% of patients.[7] In these cases, the dAVF often undergoes spontaneous regression and even resolution over time. In the presence of disabling symptoms but no retrograde CVD, use a strategy is often used that combines particle embolization for symptom palliation, and reduces the flow through the fistula followed by stereotactic radiosurgery (SRS). This strategy usually results in symptom resolution and obliteration of the fistula in more than 70% of patients (usually within a year) while preserving the patency of the involved sinus.

The presence of retrograde CVD in patients with dAVF involving a large dural sinus is often associated with progressive neurologic symptoms and disturbance of the venous drainage from the normal brain parenchyma. In these cases, a more aggressive therapy with the goal of rapid angiographic obliteration is required; this is particularly true if the venous drainage is associated with a cortical venous varix, which may increase the risk of hemorrhage.[1,7] In these cases, a transvenous approach with coil embolization of the involved sinus is preferred, which may be patent but often is not functional because it is used for the drainage of the fistula and hence arterialized.

Indirect cavernous carotid fistulas (CCF) represent a unique type of dAVF. In patients with minimal symptoms, no retrograde CVD, and normal intraocular pressure, SRS with or without transarterial particulate embolization is a safe and effective therapeutic strategy. In patients with indirect CCF and retrograde CVD and/or progressive symptoms or increased intraocular pressure, a more direct and immediate treatment is preferred, which usually involves a transvenous catheterization and occlusion of the involved area with coils and more recently Onyx in combination with coils. In these cases, the venous access to the cavernous sinus may be difficult, in which case a direct percutaneous puncture and access can be used.

Patients who present with hemorrhage also require a treatment that should be immediate and curative. The risk of rebleeding after a first hemorrhagic episode is quite high in patients with dAVF, especially if a venous varix is present along the drainage pathway.[8] Many of the patients who present with hemorrhage have dAVF in locations other than the more common transverse/sigmoid junction or the cavernous sinus. Most the fistulas presenting with hemorrhage are located in the tentorium and the anterior cranial fossa and have exclusive retrograde CVD. Onyx has dramatically improved the ability to treat effectively and safely most of the tentorial dAVF, which only a few years ago were considered almost exclusively "surgical" fistulas.[9] Transarterial Onyx embolization has a much higher chance of being effective if the posterior branch of the middle meningeal artery is one of the main feeders to the dAVF. This branch is relatively straight and allows for distal catheterization, which in turn improves the likelihood of anterograde migration of the embolic agent. For this strategy to be effective, the proximal portion of the draining vein must be completely obliterated.

Although embolization of anterior cranial fossa dAVF is feasible, surgical resection or SRS remain the preferred treatment options because of the risk of blindness from reflux of the embolic material into the ethmoidal branches of the ophthalmic artery. In the presence of aggressive clinical symptoms, surgery is also considered for those dAVF in locations other than anterior cranial fossa if embolization is not feasible or fails to obliterate the fistula completely.

With widespread utilization of axial imaging studies, a large number of dAVF are currently diagnosed in patients with minimal or no symptoms. Some of these incidental fistulas have dangerous angiographic features, including locations prone to hemorrhage (tentorial, anterior cranial fossa), presence of retrograde CVD, or an associated venous varix. In these cases, treatment in younger patients and especially in those with associated venous varices is recommended. Embolization, SRS, or a combination of both techniques is usually the main treatment strategy in these cases. Resection is reserved for those patients who fail embolization and radiosurgery. In the authors' experience, SRS is very effective in dAVF involving a large dural sinus, such as the transverse/sigmoid, the superior sagittal sinus, and indirect CCF.

CLINICAL OUTCOMES OF SRS FOR DAVF AT THE UNIVERSITY OF VIRGINIA
Demographics and Clinical Presentation

Recently the dAVF patients treated with gamma knife radiosurgery (GKRS) at the University of Virginia between 1989 and 2005 were reviewed.[10] To provide sufficient follow-up for the analysis of benefits and complications, only those patients with at least 3 years of follow-up were included. During this period of time, 55 patients with dAVF were treated. The treatment group consisted of 37 (67%) men and 18 (33%) women with an average age of 50 years. An acute change in level of consciousness was noted in 15 (27%) cases and headache was the reported by 29 (52%) patients. Seven (12%) patients reported a remote history of closed head injury. Alteration in level of consciousness was precipitated in all cases by either intracerebral hemorrhage (ICH) or spontaneous subarachnoid hemorrhage (SAH). Eleven (20%) patients had undergone craniotomy in an attempt to remove the dAVF. Endovascular therapy was undertaken in 36 (65%) patients but had proven to be unsuccessful at complete obliteration of the dAVF.

Preradiosurgical Neuro-Imaging Evaluation

Pretreatment computerized tomography (CT) or magnetic resonance image (MRI) was available in all patients. ICH was demonstrated in 20 (36%) patients, and 7 (12%) had SAH either in isolation or in addition to ICH. Hydrocephalus was found in 3 (5%) cases. Fourteen of 27 (52%) of Borden grade III patients and 2 of 12 (17%) of Borden grade II patients presented with either SAH or ICH.[11] There were 44 (80%) multihole fistulae and 39 (71%) patients demonstrated retrograde CVD. Most (27 of 55) patients with dAVF were Borden grade III, and the nidus of 26 (47%) fistulae measured between 11 and 20 mm.

GKRS Technique

The gamma knife (Elekta AB, Stockholm, Sweden) radiosurgery technique used has been previously described.[12,13] In brief, each patient underwent placement of a stereotactic frame under monitored anesthesia. Then, the patient had a thin-sliced stereotactic MRI (or CT if MRI was contraindicated) along with a cerebral angiogram. Neuro-imaging studies were imported into the gamma knife planning station and a conformal dose plan was rendered. In the authors' institutional experience, the mean prescription dose to dAVF patients was 21 Gy (range 12–33 Gy).

Clinical and Radiographic Follow-up After Radiosurgery

Follow-up MRI or CT was performed at 6-month intervals after GKRS to monitor for radiation-induced edema in the adjacent brain and for change in the volume of "flow voids" within the dAVF. If the MRI suggested angiographic obliteration, a cerebral angiogram was performed. Angiographic obliteration of the nidus defines the desired endpoint of treatment or cure. Because 3-year follow-up was not available for all, the percentage of cured patients are presented as a subset of those with 3-year angiographic follow-up (high-cure percentage) and also as a subset of all patients (low-cure percentage). All cases lost to follow-up were assumed to have been treatment failures and contribute to the low cure percentage; this percentage provided the lowest possible approximation of treatment efficacy.

Clinical Outcomes After SRS

In the series of 55 DAVF patients treated at the University of Virginia, median clinical follow-up was 11.4 years (range, 3.8–19). Reliable clinical follow-up information was available in 23 patients. Sixteen (70%) reported good or excellent health; 12 (52%) were employed in a full-time occupation, and 8 (35%) were retired. Of the retired patients, 4 were taking disability payments. Symptoms relating to the dAVF precipitated request for disability in 3 patients, whereas cardiac and pulmonary diseases were causative in a fourth patient. Twenty-two (96%) were living independently. Seventeen (74%) were no longer suffering from the preradiosurgical symptoms. Three (13%) reported persistent headaches; 2 (8.7%) had vestibular symptoms, and 1 (4%) reported blurred vision.

Obliteration Rates

Angiographic follow-up within 3 years of the GKRS was obtained in 46 of 55 patients. In 30 of these patients, arteriography demonstrated obliteration of the dAVF (**Fig. 1**). Calculation of the obliteration rate after SRS ranged between 54% (low-cure percentage) and 65% (high-cure percentage). A predictor for treatment failure was the presence of retrograde CVD on preoperative angiography.

COMPLICATIONS AND CONCERNS
Posttreatment Hemorrhage

During the latency period before obliteration, 3 patients suffered an ICH after SRS. In these 3 patients, pretreatment angiograms demonstrated retrograde CVD and were classified as Borden grade III. Fortunately, none of the patients suffered from persistent neurologic deficits as a result of the hemorrhage. In 1 of these 3, 2 consecutive bleeds occurring 2 years after radiosurgery prompted a second GKRS. Obliteration of the nidus in this particular patient was demonstrated angiographically 1 year after this second SRS. These postradiosurgical hemorrhages underscore

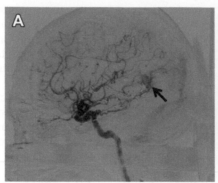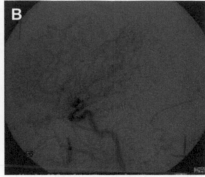

Fig. 1. Lateral cerebral angiograms of a 35-year-old woman with a severe headache and evidence of ICH at the age of 23. She underwent a craniotomy with attempted surgical clipping a complex multihole dAVF. Symptoms of headache and diplopia persisted for 12 years after surgery and the patient eventually presented with a second ICH and prolonged hospitalization. At the time of GKRS (*A*), 40 days after the second ICH, the patient complained only of intermittent headache, with angiographic evidence of persistence of flow (*arrow*) through dAVF. Angiography performed 25 months after SRS (*B*) demonstrates complete obliteration of the dAVF.

that patients remain at risk of hemorrhage until the dAVF has fully obliterated. In patients with angiographically confirmed obliteration of their dAVF, a subsequent hemorrhage has not been observed.

Neurologic Deficit After GKRS

One patient developed hemiparesis after the treatment of a tentorial dAVF. This deficit persisted until his death 4 years after SRS. No radiographic evidence of radiation-induced damage was noted on post-SRS MRI in this patient. No other patients had radiosurgically induced neurologic deficits.

Adverse Radiation Changes

MRI obtained at least 3 months after radiosurgery was available in 33 patients (63%). On T2-weighted MRI, radiation-induced change at the perimeter of the lesion was evident in 4 of 33 (12%) patients. Maximum dose and margin dose to these lesions with T2-weighted signal changes were 38 Gy and 18 Gy, respectively, which was not significantly different from patients without radiation-induced changes. In each case, adverse radiation changes were treated with corticosteroids and resolved.

OTHER CONSIDERATIONS ON DAVF RADIOSURGERY

Based on the long-term results of a large series of patients with dAVF, SRS is an effective adjuvant therapy whereby persistence of flow is found following surgery or endovascular treatment. The authors' institutional experience provides an effective obliteration range between 54% and 65% and was similar to previously published series

(**Table 1**).[10,14–25] At the Karolinska University, Soderman and colleagues[24] reported obliteration in 68% of patients. They also reported improved clinical outcome in those with naturally progressing shunts. In the experience from the University of Pittsburgh, obliteration was seen in 83% of dAVF patients who had combined SRS and embolization as compared with 67% for those with SRS alone.[25] This finding underscores the multidisciplinary approach that likely benefits many dAVF patients. They also noted that those with CCFs were more likely to achieve occlusion. Symptomatic improvement was better achieved in patients with fistulas located at the transverse-sigmoid sinus junction.

Radiosurgical doses for successful obliteration of dAVF seem comparable to those used for intracranial arteriovenous malformations (18–25 Gy). In the authors' experience, significantly improved obliteration rates were noted in Borden I lesions and, as corollary, in the absence of CVD.[10] Hence, those patients with dAVF that have the presence of persistent pial venous draining vessels seem to be less appropriate candidates for GKRS, a finding also supported by others.[24] This finding likely relates to the latency period for SRS to achieve obliteration in the setting of increased bleeding risk in patients with significant CVD.[8,11]

For those with Borden I dAVF, SRS was found to be a clinically safe procedure with all patients able to undergo treatment without subsequent intracranial hemorrhage or persistence neurologic symptoms. In all 3 cases where intracranial hemorrhage followed treatment, there was radiographic evidence of pretreatment CVD and the fistulas were designated Borden III lesions. Similarly, the one patient with persistent hemiparesis following

Table 1
Major Radiosurgery Series for Intracranial Dural Arteriovenous Fistulas

Study (Author; Publication Date)	SRS Device	Number of Patients	Imaging Follow Up (Months)	Obliteration	Post-treatment Hemorrhage
Chandler HC & Friedman WA,[14] 1993	LINAC	1	1	1	0
Lewis AI et al,[20] 1994	LINAC	7	5	3	0
Guo WY et al,[16] 1998	GK	18	15	12	0
Pollock BE et al,[21] 1999	GK	20	20	14	0
Ratliff J & Voorhies RM,[22] 1999	LINAC	1	1	1	0
Shin M et al,[23] 2000	GK	2	2	2	0
Koebbe et al,[19] 2005	GK	18	15	12	0
Soderman et al,[24] 2006	GK	49	41	28	2
Cifarelli et al,[10] 2010	GK	55	46	30	3
Yang et al,[25] 2010	GK	40	45	28	1
Jung et al,[18] 2010	GK	5	30	2	0
Hanakita et al,[17] 2012	GK	22	33	12	0
Gross et al, 2012	LINAC	9	35	8	0

treatment also had a Borden II lesion with significant pial venous drainage before SRS.

Despite advances in magnetic resonance angiography and CT angiography, angiography remains a critical component for both pretreatment and posttreatment evaluation. Also, cerebral angiography is important for accurate targeting of the dAVF at the time of radiosurgery. Certainly, the reliance on clinical symptoms for the evaluation of effectiveness of treatment is inadequate by itself and can at times be complicated by reports of spontaneous resolution of symptoms.[7] Some prior studies have incorporated both angiographic and MRI to evaluate treatment efficacy, resulting in uncertainty with respect to "cure" rate, largely due to the limited resolution of dAVF on MRI.[16] Although MR angiography is used for surveillance, cerebral angiography remains the test of choice for confirming complete obliteration of a dAVF.[26] The obvious disadvantages of angiography during follow-up imaging include procedural risk, cost, and patient discomfort. Nevertheless, weighed against the potential morbidity associated with ICH or SAH secondary to residual disease, the drawbacks of angiography are outweighed by the benefits of determining whether the dAVF is completely obliterated or, if patent, needs further intervention.

From a practical management standpoint, SRS for dAVF may also be advantageous for lesions where the risk of surgical approach is prohibitive due to deep location or where the vascular architecture exceeds the capacity of endovascular catheter access. As endovascular therapy remains the mainstay of treatment for dAVF, it is unlikely that SRS will eclipse neuro-interventional procedures. Nevertheless, SRS will remain an important and effective treatment for many patients with intracranial dAVF.

SUMMARY

Stereotactic radiosurgery is a safe and effective therapy for dAVF, for patients with residual lesions after prior resection or endovascular treatment, and in some cases as an upfront treatment. Patients without CVD are more likely to demonstrate obliteration without significant risk of hemorrhage during the latency period or neurologic deficit following SRS.

REFERENCES

1. Awad IA, Little JR, Akarawi WP, et al. Intracranial dural arteriovenous malformations: factors predisposing to an aggressive neurological course. J Neurosurg 1990;72:839–50.
2. Hai J, Ding M, Guo Z, et al. A new rat model of chronic cerebral hypoperfusion associated with arteriovenous malformations. J Neurosurg 2002;97: 1198–202.
3. Terada T, Higashida RT, Halbach VV, et al. Development of acquired arteriovenous fistulas in rats due to venous hypertension. J Neurosurg 1994;80: 884–9.

4. Uranishi R, Nakase H, Sakaki T. Expression of angiogenic growth factors in dural arteriovenous fistula. J Neurosurg 1999;91:781–6.

5. Kojima T, Miyachi S, Sahara Y, et al. The relationship between venous hypertension and expression of vascular endothelial growth factor: hemodynamic and immunohistochemical examinations in a rat venous hypertension model. Surg Neurol 2007;68: 277–84.

6. van Dijk JM, terBrugge KG, Willinsky RA, et al. Clinical course of cranial dural arteriovenous fistulas with long-term persistent cortical venous reflux. Stroke 2002;33:1233–6.

7. Brown RD Jr, Wiebers DO, Nichols DA. Intracranial dural arteriovenous fistulae: angiographic predictors of intracranial hemorrhage and clinical outcome in nonsurgical patients. J Neurosurg 1994;81:531–8.

8. Duffau H, Lopes M, Janosevic V, et al. Early rebleeding from intracranial dural arteriovenous fistulas: report of 20 cases and review of the literature. J Neurosurg 1999;90:78–84.

9. Puffer RC, Daniels DJ, Kallmes DF, et al. Curative Onyx embolization of tentorial dural arteriovenous fistulas. Neurosurg Focus 2012;32:E4.

10. Cifarelli CP, Kaptain G, Yen CP, et al. Gamma Knife radiosurgery for dural arteriovenous fistulas. Neurosurgery 2010;67(5):1230–5.

11. Borden JA, Wu JK, Shucart WA. A proposed classification for spinal and cranial dural arteriovenous fistulous malformations and implications for treatment. J Neurosurg 1995;82:166–79.

12. Cheng CH, Crowley RW, Yen CP, et al. Gamma Knife surgery for basal ganglia and thalamic arteriovenous malformations. J Neurosurg 2012;116: 899–908.

13. Yen CP, Steiner L. Gamma knife surgery for brainstem arteriovenous malformations. World Neurosurg 2011;76:87–95.

14. Chandler HC Jr, Friedman WA. Successful radiosurgical treatment of a dural arteriovenous malformation: case report. Neurosurgery 1993;33:139–42.

15. Gross BA, Ropper AE, Popp AJ, et al. Stereotactic radiosurgery for cerebral dural arteriovenous fistulas. Neurosurg Focus 2012;32(5):E18.

16. Guo WY, Pan DH, Wu HM, et al. Radiosurgery as a treatment alternative for dural arteriovenous fistulas of the cavernous sinus. AJNR Am J Neuroradiol 1998;19:1081–7.

17. Hanakita S, Koga T, Shin M, et al. Role of Gamma Knife surgery in the treatment of intracranial dural arteriovenous fistulas. J Neurosurg 2012; 117(Suppl):158–63.

18. Jung HH, Chang JH, Whang K, et al. Gamma Knife surgery for low-flow cavernous sinus dural arteriovenous fistulas. J Neurosurg 2010; 113(Suppl):21–7.

19. Koebbe CJ, Singhal D, Sheehan J, et al. Radiosurgery for dural arteriovenous fistulas. Surg Neurol 2005;64:392–8.

20. Lewis AI, Tomsick TA, Tew JM Jr. Management of tentorial arteriovenous malformations: transarterial embolization combined with stereotactic radiation or surgery. J Neurosurg 1994;81:851–9.

21. Pollock BE, Nichols DA, Garrity JA, et al. Stereotactic radiosurgery and particulate embolization for cavernous sinus dural arteriovenous fistulae. Neurosurgery 1999;45:459–67.

22. Ratliff J, Voorhies RM. Arteriovenous fistula with associated aneurysms coexisting with dural arteriovenous malformation of the anterior inferior falx. Case report and review of the literature. J Neurosurg 1999;91:303–7.

23. Shin M, Kurita H, Tago M, et al. Stereotactic radiosurgery for tentorial dural arteriovenous fistulae draining into the vein of Galen: report of two cases. Neurosurgery 2000;46:730–4.

24. Soderman M, Edner G, Ericson K, et al. Gamma knife surgery for dural arteriovenous shunts: 25 years of experience. J Neurosurg 2006;104:867–75.

25. Yang HC, Kano H, Kondziolka D, et al. Stereotactic radiosurgery with or without embolization for intracranial dural arteriovenous fistulas. Neurosurgery 2010;67:1276–83.

26. Meckel S, Maier M, Ruiz DS, et al. MR angiography of dural arteriovenous fistulas: diagnosis and follow-up after treatment using a time-resolved 3D contrast-enhanced technique. AJNR Am J Neuroradiol 2007;28:877–84.

Stereotactic Radiosurgery for Brain Metastases

Toru Serizawa, MD, PhD[a],*, Yoshinori Higuchi, MD, PhD[b],
Osamu Nagano, MD, PhD[c]

KEYWORDS

- Stereotactic radiosurgery • Gamma Knife radiosurgery • Brain metastases
- Whole-brain radiation therapy

KEY POINTS

- Good indications for Gamma Knife (Elekta AB, Stockholm, Sweden) radiosurgery (GKS) are (1) volume of the largest tumor less than 10 cm^3, (2) a Karnofsky performance status score of 70 or more, (3) no magnetic resonance imaging evidence of cerebrospinal fluid dissemination, (4) total tumor volume of 15 cm^3 or less, and (5) tumor number of 10 or less.
- The local tumor control rates at 1 year were 84.8% for less than 1 cm^3, 86.0% for 1 to 4 cm^3, 76.2% for 4 to 10 cm^3, and 55.3% for more than 10 cm^3 lesions. Two-staged or 3-staged GKS may be useful for large tumors.
- A total skull absorbed energy dose of 10J is the limitation, regardless of tumor number and size, in GKS. Within these limits, 25 tiny, 10 small, or 3 to 4 medium-sized lesions can be safely treated.
- A prospective, multi-institutional trial (UMIN ID 0000001812) is ongoing to assess the noninferiority, in terms of survival period, of GKS alone for treating patients with 5 to 10 brain metastases as compared with those with 2 to 4.

INTRODUCTION

Whole-brain radiation therapy (WBRT), with or without surgery, has been the gold standard of treatment of patients with brain metastases. Stereotactic radiosurgery (SRS) offers many benefits as compared with surgery and/or WBRT because the procedures are minimally invasive and can also be performed as one-day treatment. In the same session, SRS may be used to treat multiple lesions. Furthermore, SRS can be used for disparate or eloquent locations not conducive to open surgical approaches by delivering higher radiation doses. SRS also avoids leukoencephalopathy, which develops in some patients after WBRT.[1–3]

Surgical resection of a single brain metastasis has been shown to improve tumor control and prolong survival, particularly when combined with WBRT.[4,5] However, surgical resection may be contraindicated in most patients because of poor general condition or inaccessible locations.[6] For more than 2 decades, SRS has provided patients who have metastatic brain tumors with a local treatment alternative to surgery. Studies have shown that SRS is very effective in controlling brain metastases, preventing neurologic death, and maintaining good activities of daily living.[7–15] Moreover, SRS is minimally invasive and can be performed with a short hospitalization, which are important considerations for quality of life and health care economics as compared with surgery.[16,17] Another treatment option for brain metastases, chemotherapy, has been considered

Disclosures: The authors have nothing to disclose.
[a] Tokyo Gamma Unit Center, Tsukiji Neurological Clinic, 1-9-9 Tsukiji, Chuo-ku, Tokyo, Japan; [b] Department of Neurological Surgery, Chiba University Graduate School of Medicine, Chiba, Japan; [c] Gamma Knife House, Chiba Cardiovascular Center, Ichihara, Japan
* Corresponding author.
E-mail address: gamma-knife.serizawa@nifty.com

Neurosurg Clin N Am 24 (2013) 597–603
http://dx.doi.org/10.1016/j.nec.2013.05.007
1042-3680/13/$ – see front matter © 2013 Elsevier Inc. All rights reserved.

ineffective because of poor penetration across the blood-brain barrier. However, cytotoxic chemotherapy is potentially effective, particularly for chemosensitive tumor types, such as small cell lung cancer and breast cancer. Recently, molecular targeting agents, such as tyrosine kinase inhibitors, which target epidermal growth receptor (EGFR) and human epidermal growth factor 2 (HER2), have been shown to be very effective for brain metastases from lung cancer with the EGFR mutation or breast cancer overexpressing HER2. Under such circumstances, these molecular targeting agents might be effective even in cases with cerebral and/or cerebrospinal small fluid (CSF) dissemination not receiving WBRT.[18]

In this article, the authors present the results of Gamma Knife (Elekta AB, Stockholm, Sweden) radiosurgery (GKS) for brain metastases based on their retrospective review of 2645 brain metastasis cases treated during a 15-year period, focusing on 5 prognostic factors.

RADIOSURGICAL TECHNIQUE

Patient characteristics are summarized in **Table 1**. All aspects of patient selection, dose planning, dose selection, performing GKS, and collecting follow-up data, were undertaken by the first author (T.S.). All patients were treated according to the same protocol, as reported previously.[13] At the initial treatment, all lesions were irradiated with GKS without up-front WBRT. In some cases with tumor volumes exceeding 10 cm^3, staged GKS was chosen.[19] In all patients with a total tumor volume exceeding 15 cm^3 and/or tumor numbers greater than 25, the GKS procedures were divided into 2 or 3 sessions to ensure a total skull absorbed energy (TSAE) of less than 10 J, thereby preventing acute brain swelling.[20] New distant lesions, detected by gadolinium-enhanced magnetic resonance imaging (MRI) performed every 2 to 3 months, were treated mainly with GKS and sometimes with WBRT, only if cerebral and/or CSF dissemination was detected. The standard prescribed dose at the tumor periphery of 20 Gy was changed depending on the primary cancer, physical status, tumor location, and tumor volume (including in the staged GKS cases).

PROGNOSTIC FACTORS
Tumor Size

Fig. 1 demonstrates tumor progression-free survival curves according to the tumor volume treated with GKS in 2374 lesions, with the largest volume selected in each case (excluding 271 lesions treated using the staged GKS). Tumor

Table 1
Patient characteristics

Characteristics	Covariates	Total
Case number	Total	2645
Age (y)	Median (min-max)	65 (27–96)
Gender	Male	1583 (59.8%)
	Female	1062 (40.2%)
Extracranial disease	Controlled	326 (12.3%)
	Active	2319 (87.7%)
Pretreatment KPS score	Median (min-max)	100 (50–100)
Primary organ	Lung	1729 (65.4%)
	GI-tract	332 (12.5%)
	Breast	290 (11.0%)
	Urogenital	167 (6.3%)
	Others	127 (4.8%)
Number of brain lesions	Median (min-max)	3 (1–100)
	Single	728 (27.5%)
	2–4	885 (33.5%)
	5–10	581 (22.0%)
	>10	451 (17.1%)
Maximum lesion volume (cm^3)	Median (min-max)	2.8 (0.1–72.5)
Total tumor volume (cm^3)	Median (min-max)	4.5 (0.1–100.0)
Neurologic symptoms	Yes	1434 (54.2%)
	No	1211 (45.8%)
RTOG-RPA classification	Class I	142 (5.4%)
	Class II	2150 (81.3%)
	Class III	353 (13.3%)

Abbreviations: GI, gastrointestinal; KPS, Karnofsky performance status; min, minimum; max, maximum; RPA, recursive partitioning analysis; RTOG, Radiation Therapy Oncology Group.

volumes were divided into 4 groups: tiny (<1 cm^3), small (1–4 cm^3), medium (4–10 cm^3), and large (>10 cm^3). Control of GKS-treated lesions was defined as the lack of any significant increase in tumor diameter (<20%). The tumor control rates at 1 year were 84.8% for 794 tiny tumors (mean dose, 21.2 Gy), 86.0% for 854 small tumors (mean dose, 20.6 Gy), 76.2% for 588 medium-sized tumors (mean dose, 19.6 Gy), and 55.3% for 238 large tumors (mean dose, 17.2 Gy). The differences in tumor control were statistically significant between all pairs of adjacent tumor volume groups (tiny vs small, $P<.0001$; small vs medium, $P = .0002$; medium vs large, $P = .0002$). These results suggest that for large tumors, staged GKS should be

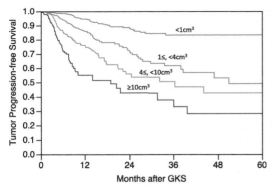

Fig. 1. Tumor progression-free survival curves according to tumor volume. The tumor control rates at 1 year were 84.8% for 794 tiny tumors (<1 cm³, *orange*, mean prescribed dose, 21.2 Gy), 86.0% for 854 small tumors (1–4 cm³, *blue*, 20.6 Gy), 76.2% for 588 medium tumors (4–10 cm³, *green*, 19.6 Gy), and 55.3% for 238 large tumors (>10 cm³, *red*, 17.2 Gy). The differences were statistically significant between all pairs of adjacent groups (tiny vs small, *P*<.0001; small vs medium-sized, *P* = .0002; medium-sized vs large, *P* = .0002).

considered, depending on life expectancy, as the authors previously proposed.[19]

Karnofsky Performance Score

Gaspar proposed the recursive partitioning analysis (RPA) system for predicting the outcomes of patients with brain metastasis[21] treated with WBRT according to the Karnofsky performance scale (KPS) score,[22] age, primary tumor control, and extracranial metastases. **Fig. 2** shows the overall survival (OS) curves according to the RPA class. Median survival time (MST) was 22.8 months

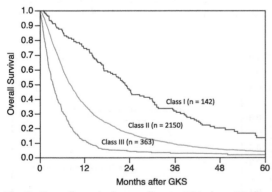

Fig. 2. Overall survival according to RPA class. Median survival time was 22.8 months in class I (142 cases, indicated in *red*), 8.3 in class II (2150 cases, indicated in *green*), and 3.5 in class III (363 cases, indicated in *blue*). There were significant differences between both pairs of adjacent classes (*P*<.0001).

in class I (n = 142), 8.3 in class II (n = 2150), and 3.5 in class III (n = 363). There were significant differences between both pairs of adjacent classes (*P*<.0001). Patients in RPA class III, which means KPS score less than 70%, seemed to not be good candidates for GKS. However, even for patients in class III, with severe neurologic symptoms, such as hemiparesis, cerebellar ataxia, dizziness, and so on, GKS should definitely be considered. Other grading systems, such as the Score Index for SRS,[23] Basic Score for Brain Metastases,[24] Graded Prognostic Assessment,[25] and Modified RPA,[26] have been proposed for predicting the survival of patients with brain metastasis; these systems are also useful for deciding indications.

CSF Dissemination

Neurologic death (**Fig. 3**A) and neurologic deterioration (see **Fig. 3**B) for patients with and without MRI evidence of CSF dissemination are shown in **Fig. 3**. Neurologic death was defined as death from any expression of intracranial metastases (tumor recurrence, carcinomatous meningitis, cerebral dissemination) and neurologic deterioration as impaired neurologic status (KPS <70). CSF dissemination is defined as enhancement in the brain sulci, ventricular wall, and basal cistern on dose-planning MRI, which is taken at a 2-mm thickness without gaps using double-dose gadolinium enhancement. The difference was statistically significant (*P*<.0001) in terms of both neurologic death and neurologic deterioration. These data were not corrected with competing risk analysis, so the absolute values are only advisory. In general, CSF dissemination is a contraindication for SRS alone.[16,17] If MRI findings of CSF dissemination are present on the dose-planning images, treatment combining WBRT and/or small molecular targeting agents with GKS should be considered.

Total Tumor Volume

The authors have advocated the 10J-TSAE concept, based on tumor number and size limitations in a single GKS for safety reasons, as already reported.[20] This 10J-TSAE is roughly equivalent to 3 Gy of the mean whole-brain radiation. Within these limits, the authors assume that 25 tiny, 10 small, or 4 medium-sized lesions, if the tumors are approximately the same size and diffusely located in the brain, can be safely treated. The 10J-TSAE is estimated almost the same irradiation dose to 15 cm³ total tumor volume with a prescribed dose of 20 to 22 Gy. Rates of neurologic death (**Fig. 4**A) and neurologic deterioration (see **Fig. 4**B) were significantly higher in cases with

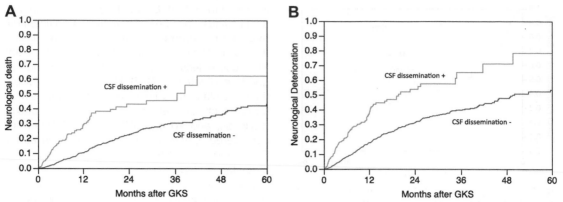

Fig. 3. Neurologic death (*A*) and neurologic deterioration (*B*) in patients with and without MRI evidence of CSF dissemination are shown. The difference was statistically significant (*P*<.0001).

more than 15 cm³ total tumor volume as compared with those with 15 cm³ or less. The differences were significant (both *P*<.0001). These results suggest that cases with total tumor volumes greater than 15 cm³ are not good candidates for GKS alone for safety reasons and also because of poor outcomes. The total tumor volume and the presence of CSF dissemination are more important factors than tumor number in determining the treatment strategy for brain metastasis. For cases with total tumor volumes greater than 15 cm³, combined WBRT, staged or multisession GKS and stereotactic radiotherapy using the linear particle accelerator system should be considered depending on patients' preferences, intracranial disease status, physical status, and the radiation sensitivity of the primary cancer.

Number of Tumors

Aoyama and colleagues[27] published the results of the Japanese Radiation Oncology Study Group 99-1 in 2006, showing the efficacy of SRS alone for patients with 1 to 4 brain metastases. However, the authors often find additional tiny lesions on dose-planning MRI using double-dose gadolinium enhancement with thin slices. How many brain metastases are acceptable for GKS alone treatment? **Fig. 5**A shows OS curves according to the tumor number. The authors divided patients into 4 groups based on tumor number: single in 728 cases, 2 to 4 in 885, 5 to 10 in 581, and more than 10 in 451. The MSTs were 10.0, 7.7, 6.9, and 5.9 months for cases with single, 2 to 4, 5 to 10, and more than 10 tumors, respectively. There were statistically significant differences between all pairs of adjacent tumor number groups (single vs 2–4, *P*<.0001; 2–4 vs 5–10, *P* = .0054; 5–10 vs >10, *P* = .0127). Focusing on neurologic death (see **Fig. 5**B) and deterioration (see **Fig. 5**C), the results of groups with 2 to 4 and 5 to 10 brain metastases were essentially the same. These results suggested that patients with 5 to 10 brain metastases are acceptable candidates for GKS alone, based on comparison with patients with 2 to 4 lesions. **Fig. 5**D demonstrates

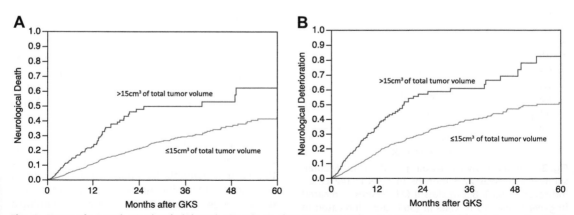

Fig. 4. Rates of neurologic death (*A*) and neurologic deterioration (*B*) were significantly higher in cases with a total tumor volume greater than 15 cm³. The differences were significant (both *P*<.0001).

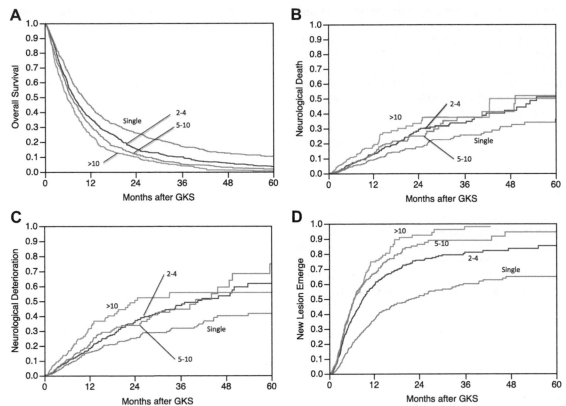

Fig. 5. OS, neurologic death, neurologic deterioration, and emergence of new distant lesions according to number of tumors at the time of GKS. (*A*) OS curves according to tumor number. Median survival time was 10.0, 7.7, 6.9, and 5.9 months for cases with 1 tumor (n = 428), 2 to 4 tumors (n = 885), 5 to 10 tumors (n = 581), and more than 10 tumors (n = 451), respectively. There were statistically significant differences between all pairs of adjacent tumor number groups (1 vs 2–4, *P*<.0001; 2–4 vs 5–10, *P* = .0054; 5–10 vs >10, *P* = .0127). (*B*) Neurologic death. (*C*) Neurologic deterioration. The results of groups with 2 to 4 and 5 to 10 brain metastases were nearly the same. (*D*) New distant lesion emergence according to tumor number. There were significant differences between the group with 1 tumor and the group with 2 to 4 tumors (*P*<.0001) as well as between the group with 2 to 4 tumors and the group with 5 to 10 tumors (*P* = .0005), but the incidence differed minimally between the group with 5 to 10 tumors and the group with more than 10 tumors (*P* = .23).

new distant tumor formation according to the number of tumors at the time of GKS. The higher the tumor number, the more frequently new lesions emerged. There were significant differences between single and 2 to 4 (*P*<.0001) as well as between 2 to 4 and 5 to 10 lesions (*P* = .0005), but the incidences in patients with 5 to 10 and more than 10 were nearly equal (*P* = .23). GKS alone should be performed when follow-up MRI and salvage GKS are available.

It is anticipated that the efficacy of GKS alone for up to 10 brain metastases will be established by the JLGK0901 study (UMIN ID 0000001812), which is a prospective multi-institute trial currently being conducted in Japan.[28–30] This study aims to show the noninferiority of GKS for patients with 5 to 10 brain metastases as compared with those with 2 to 4 tumors in terms of OS.

COMPLICATIONS AND CONCERNS

Complications of GKS for brain metastases in the acute (within 3 days) and subacute (3 weeks) phases are relatively rare. Tumor bleeding, acute brain swelling, and convulsions may occur. The most common complication is regrowth of GKS-treated lesions (enlargement of enhanced lesions with surrounding edema). This phenomenon, called *radiation injury*, often occurs around 6 to 12 months after GKS. Radiation injury consists of necrosis of the tumor and normal brain tissue combined with recurrent viable tumor cells. Differentiating between radiation injury and tumor recurrence is often difficult using only enhanced MRI because the lesion has mixed components and may change over time. The efficacies of magnetic resonance spectroscopy, single photon emission computerized tomography, and positron emission tomography have been reported.[31-33]

Another concern after GKS is the salvage treatment of new distant lesions. The authors' treatment strategy is to avoid prophylactic WBRT at the initial treatment. If new distant lesions are detected on follow-up MRI conducted every 2 to 3 months, salvage GKS is considered. When CSF dissemination is detected, salvage WBRT is performed depending on the patients' KPS and systemic disease status.

SUMMARY

Based on the authors' experience with GKS for brain metastases, good indications for GKS alone are (1) volume of the largest tumor less than 10 cm^3, (2) a KPS score of 70 or more, (3) no MRI evidence of carcinomatous meningitis, (4) total tumor volume of 15 cm^3 or less, and (5) total tumor number of 10 or less. New distant lesions are generally well controlled with GKS salvage treatment. However, careful observation with enhanced MRI and appropriate salvage treatments are needed to maximize patient survival.

REFERENCES

1. Asai A, Matsutani M, Kohno T, et al. Subacute brain atrophy after irradiation therapy for malignant brain tumor. Cancer 1989;63:1962–74.

2. DeAngelis LM, Delattre JY, Posner JB. Radiation-induced dementia in patients cured of brain metastases. Neurology 1989;39:789–96.

3. Chan E, Wefel J, Hess K, et al. Neurocognition in patients with brain metastases treated radiosurgery or radiosurgery plus whole-brain irradiation: a randomized controlled trial. Lancet Oncol 2009;5:1–8.

4. Patchell RA, Tibbs PA, Regine WF, et al. Postoperative radiotherapy in treatment of single metastases to the brain: a randomized trial. JAMA 1998;280: 1485–9.

5. Patchell RA, Tibbs PA, Walsh JW, et al. A randomized trial of surgery in the treatment of single metastases to the brain. N Engl J Med 1990;322: 494–500.

6. Sawaya R, Bindal RK, Lang FF, et al, editors. Metastatic brain tumors. 2nd edition. New York: Churchill Livingstone; 2001.

7. Pirzkall A, Debus J, Lohr F, et al. Radiosurgery alone or in combination with whole-brain radiotherapy for brain metastases. J Clin Oncol 1998;16:3563–9.

8. Kondziolka D, Patel A, Lunsford LD, et al. Stereotactic radiosurgery plus whole brain radiotherapy versus radiotherapy alone for patients with multiple brain metastases. Int J Radiat Oncol Biol Phys 1999;45:427–34.

9. Serizawa T, Iuchi T, Ono J, et al. Gamma knife treatment for multiple metastatic brain tumors compared with whole-brain radiation therapy. J Neurosurg 2000;93:32–6.

10. Shaw E, Scott C, Souhami L, et al. Single dose radiosurgical treatment of recurrent previously irradiated primary brain tumors and brain metastases. Int J Radiat Oncol Biol Phys 2000;47:291–8.

11. Serizawa T, Ono J, Iuchi T, et al. Gamma knife radiosurgery for metastatic brain tumors from lung cancer. Comparison between small cell cancer and non-small cell cancer. J Neurosurg 2002;97(Suppl 5):484–8.

12. Lutterbach J, Cyron D, Henne K, et al. Radiosurgery followed by planned observation in patients with one to three brain metastases. Neurosurgery 2003;52: 1066–73.

13. Serizawa T, Higuchi Y, Ono J, et al. Gamma knife surgery for metastatic brain tumor without prophylactic whole brain radiation therapy: results in 1000 consecutive cases. J Neurosurg 2006;105:86–90.

14. Serizawa T, Yamamoto M, Nagano O, et al. Gamma knife surgery for metastatic brain tumors. A 2-institute study in Japan. J Neurosurg 2008;109:118–21.

15. Rades D, Bohlen G, Pluemer A, et al. Stereotactic radiosurgery alone versus resection plus whole-brain radiotherapy for 1 or 2 brain metastases in recursive partitioning analysis class 1 and 2 patients. Cancer 2007;109:2515–21.

16. Mehta M, Noyes W, Craig B, et al. A cost-effectiveness and cost-utility analysis of radiosurgery vs. resection for single-brain metastases. Int J Radiat Oncol Biol Phys 1997;39:445–54.

17. Mehta MP, Rozental JM, Levin AB, et al. Defining the role of radiosurgery in the management of brain metastases. Int J Radiat Oncol Biol Phys 1992;24: 619–25.

18. Lee SH. Role of chemotherapy on brain metastasis. Prog Neurol Surg 2012;25:110–4.

19. Higuchi Y, Serizawa T, Nagano O, et al. Three-staged stereotactic radiotherapy without whole brain irradiation for large metastatic brain tumors. Int J Radiat Oncol Biol Phys 2009;74:1543–8.

20. Serizawa T, Saeki N, Higuchi Y, et al. Gamma knife surgery for brain metastases: indications for and limitations of a local treatment protocol. Acta Neurochir (Wien) 2005;147:721–6.

21. Gaspar L, Scott C, Rotman M, et al. Recursive partitioning analysis (RPA) of prognostic factors in three Radiation Therapy Oncology Group (RTOG) brain metastases trials. Int J Radiat Oncol Biol Phys 1997;37:745–51.

22. Karnofsky DA, Buechenal JH. The clinical evaluation of chemotherapeutic agents in cancer. In: MacLeod CM, editor. Evaluation of chemotherapeutic agents. New York: Columbia Univ Press; 1949. p. 191–205.

23. Weltman E, Salvajoli JV, Brandt RA, et al. Radiosurgery for brain metastases: a score index for predicting prognosis. Int J Radiat Oncol Biol Phys 2000;46:1155–61.

24. Lorenzoni J, Devriendt D, Massager N, et al. Radiosurgery for treatment of brain metastases: Estimation of patient eligibility using three stratification systems. Int J Radiat Oncol Biol Phys 2004;60:218–24.

25. Sperduto PW, Berkey B, Gasper LE, et al. A new prognostic index and comparison to three other indices for patients with brain metastases: an analysis of 1,960 patients in the RTOG database. Int J Radiat Oncol Biol Phys 2008;70:510–4.

26. Yamamoto M, Serizawa T, Sato Y, et al. Validity of two recently-proposed prognostic grading indices for lung, gastro-intestinal, breast and renal cell cancer patients with radiosurgically-treated brain metastases. J Neurooncol 2013;111:327–35.

27. Aoyama H, Shirato H, Tago M, et al. Stereotactic radiosurgery plus whole brain radiation therapy vs. stereotactic radiosurgery alone for treatment of brain metastases: a randomized controlled trial. JAMA 2006;295:2483–91.

28. Serizawa T, Hirai T, Nagano O, et al. Gamma knife surgery for 1-10 brain metastases without prophylactic whole-brain radiation therapy: analysis of cases meeting the Japanese prospective multi-institute study (JLGK0901) inclusion criteria. J Neurooncol 2010;98:163–7.

29. Serizawa T, Yamamoto M, Sato Y, et al. Gamma knife surgery as sole treatment for multiple brain metastases: 2-center retrospective review of 1508 cases meeting the inclusion criteria of the JLGK0901 multi-institutional prospective study. J Neurosurg 2010;113:48–52.

30. Serizawa T, Higuchi Y, Nagano O, et al. Analysis of 2000 cases treated with gamma knife surgery: validating eligibility criteria for a prospective multi-institutional study of stereotactic radiosurgery alone for treatment of patients with 1-10 brain metastases (JLGK0901) in Japan. Journal of Radiosurgery and SBRT 2012;2:19–27.

31. Serizawa T, Saeki N, Higuchi Y, et al. Diagnostic value of thallium-201 chloride single-photon emission computerized tomography in differentiating tumor recurrence from radiation injury after gamma surgery for metastatic brain tumors. J Neurosurg 2005;102:266–71.

32. Kano H, Kondziolka D, Lobato-Polo J, et al. T1/T2 matching to differentiate tumor growth from radiation effects after stereotactic radiosurgery. Neurosurgery 2010;66:486–91.

33. Belohlávek O, Simonová G, Kantorová I, et al. Brain metastases after stereotactic radiosurgery using the Leksell gamma knife: can FDG PET help to differentiate radionecrosis from tumour progression? Eur J Nucl Med Mol Imaging 2003;30:96–100.

Stereotactic Radiosurgery for Intracranial Gliomas

Shota Tanaka, MD*, Masahiro Shin, MD, PhD,
Akitake Mukasa, MD, PhD, Shunya Hanakita, MD,
Kuniaki Saito, MD, Tomoyuki Koga, MD, PhD,
Nobuhito Saito, MD, PhD

KEYWORDS

- Stereotactic radiosurgery • Glioblastoma • Low-grade glioma • Radiation necrosis • Bevacizumab

KEY POINTS

- Despite numerous retrospective and prospective studies showing the benefit of stereotactic radiosurgery (SRS) in the treatment of newly diagnosed and recurrent high-grade gliomas, the only randomized trial (RTOG 93-05) failed to demonstrate survival benefit of SRS when added to postoperative adjuvant radiotherapy and chemotherapy for newly diagnosed glioblastoma.
- The combination of bevacizumab, a monoclonal antibody against vascular endothelial growth factor, and SRS seems promising and may reduce the high rate of local recurrence and risk of radiation necrosis.
- Only several small retrospective studies are available in the literature on SRS for low-grade glioma, warranting prospective studies to assess its long-term efficacy and safety in this more benign disease.

INTRODUCTION

Gliomas are one of the most common primary brain tumors along with meningioma, affecting approximately 6 per 100,000 person-years in the United States.[1] It mainly comprises astrocytic tumors and oligodendroglial tumors of various histopathological grades; glioblastoma represents a subtype of the highest grade (World Health Organization [WHO] grade 4), characterized with its aggressiveness in tumor behavior and the dismal prognosis despite the aggressive treatment with resection followed by fractionated radiotherapy and temozolomide.

Glioblastoma is known to infiltrate extensively into the normal brain, which often prevents us from surgically resecting the tumor completely, hence becoming the ground for "involved-field" external beam radiotherapy covering the tumor area as well as a 2- to 2.5-cm margin around it. It has been intuitively thought that stereotactic radiosurgery (SRS) characterized with its steep dose falloff would be only indicated in selected cases of this infiltrative, malignant neoplasm. Nevertheless, with the widespread use of SRS for various types of brain tumors in recent years, it has been extensively investigated in the treatment of glioblastoma as well. In fact, SRS can be administered as a single session or in a small number of fractions on an outpatient basis, which would impact quality of life of the affected patients favorably, especially given the guarded prognosis of this disease. SRS may be suitable for some low-grade gliomas because they tend to form discrete masses in contrast to glioblastoma, and indeed, it has been applied successfully in some cases.

Disclosures: The authors have nothing to disclose.
Department of Neurosurgery, The University of Tokyo Hospital, 7-3-1 Hongo, Bunkyo-ku, Tokyo 113-8655, Japan
* Corresponding author.
E-mail address: tanakas-tky@alumni.mayo.edu

Neurosurg Clin N Am 24 (2013) 605–612
http://dx.doi.org/10.1016/j.nec.2013.05.010
1042-3680/13/$ – see front matter © 2013 Elsevier Inc. All rights reserved.

Little is definitely known, however, regarding the long-term efficacy and safety of SRS for such benign tumors.

Here an overview of SRS treatment of glioblastoma as well as other types of glioma is presented and its efficacy in terms of tumor control and patient survival is discussed. Also provided are the future perspectives of SRS in the treatment of glioma.

RADIOSURGERY FOR NEWLY DIAGNOSED GLIOBLASTOMA

Glioblastoma almost inevitably recurs despite the aggressive combined therapies, which urges us to maximize the initial treatments to keep the tumor at bay longer. Given the high frequency of local recurrence of glioblastoma,[2,3] additional radiation seems to offer a reasonable benefit. Although some reports argue for up-dosing fractionated radiotherapy,[4] most reports would favor for a boost with SRS, trying to minimize radiation injury to the adjacent normal brain. Historically, many retrospective studies claimed feasibility and apparent efficacy of the combined radiation,[5–8] which was supported by some,[9,10] but not all,[8,11] prospective studies. A prospective study conducted by Mehta and colleagues[10] reported a 2-year survival rate of 28% in 31 patients with newly diagnosed glioblastoma treated with the conventional radiotherapy with an SRS boost, which was significantly superior to 9.7% in the previous Radiation Therapy Oncology Group (RTOG) study patients. It is noteworthy that this "boost" approach is subject to selection bias given that it could potentially select out patients who improved or remained stable after completion of fractionated radiotherapy.[12]

Subsequently, a multicenter randomized phase III trial (RTOG 93-05) was undertaken to assess the efficacy of SRS followed by the standard adjuvant radiochemotherapy for newly diagnosed glioblastoma.[13] A total of 203 patients were randomly assigned either to SRS followed by radiotherapy and carmustine or to radiotherapy and carmustine alone, and the median overall survival (OS) was 13.5 months for the SRS group and 13.6 months for the standard treatment group at a median follow-up of 61 months. The study failed to demonstrate the improved patient survival with the combined radiation. Of note, it must be interpreted with caution for the following reasons: (1) SRS was administered before fractionated radiotherapy instead of as a boost following radiotherapy, which has become the more common practice; and (2) carmustine was used for chemotherapy because the study predated the use of temozolomide, the current standard chemotherapy agent for newly diagnosed glioblastoma. Nonetheless, the lack of survival benefit in this randomized trial reduced the enthusiasm about SRS for newly diagnosed glioblastoma, and thus, no additional clinical trials have been performed.

RADIOSURGERY FOR RECURRENT HIGH-GRADE GLIOMA

The management of a patient with glioblastoma becomes more challenging when the tumor recurs. Bevacizumab, a humanized monoclonal antibody against vascular endothelial growth factor, seems to improve progression-free survival (PFS), although its overall survival benefit is less convincing.[14,15] In addition, bevacizumab may enhance the infiltrative nature of the tumor in the form of nonenhancing progression and also increase the risk of distant recurrence,[16,17] making further treatment even more difficult. SRS has been accepted as a salvage therapy option along with fractionated stereotactic radiotherapy[18]; many studies have indicated the efficacy of SRS for recurrent glioblastoma or high-grade glioma (**Table 1**).[19–24] A prospective cohort study by Kong and colleagues[19] reported on 65 patients with recurrent glioblastoma and 49 patients with recurrent anaplastic astrocytoma that the median PFS from SRS was 4.6 and 8.6 months and the median OS from SRS was 13 and 26 months, respectively. Compared with their historical controls, SRS significantly prolonged survival in patients with recurrent glioblastoma. Of note, SRS was only indicated for tumors measuring ≤3 cm in maximal dimension, suggesting a potential selection bias. In addition, the historical controls might not have been well matched given the sequential chronologic order (historical controls followed by study patients) of treatment. Chemotherapy with temozolomide was administered along with SRS in some studies, expecting its possible radiosensitization effect.[20] With the lack of prospective studies, definitive conclusion regarding the additive effect of temozolomide is yet to be drawn.

FUTURE DIRECTIONS OF RADIOSURGERY FOR HIGH-GRADE GLIOMA

Optimal SRS—including treatment regimens for high-grade glioma—remains elusive and several novel approaches have been undertaken aiming at better outcome with less complication. Recently, there has been renewed enthusiasm in SRS treatment of glioblastoma since the promising results of SRS in conjunction with

Table 1
Treatment characteristics and patient survival in selected recent series of SRS for recurrent maligant glioma

Series	Pathology	No. of Patients	Modality	Median Dose (Gy)	Median Volume (mL)	Median Progression-Free Survival from SRS (mo)	Median Overall Survival from SRS (mo)
Kong et al,[19] 2008	GBM/AA, AOA	65/49	GKRS	16	10.6	4.6/8.6	13/26
Patel et al,[21] 2009	GBM	26/10	GKRS/HSRT	18/36 (6 fractions)	10.4/51.1	N/A	8.5/7.4
Pouratian et al,[23] 2009	GBM	26	GKRS	6	21.3	7.1	9.4
Villavicencio et al,[25] 2009	GBM	26	CyberKnife	20 (2 fractions)	7	N/A	7
Elliott et al,[24] 2010	GBM/AA/AOA	16/5/5	GKRS	15/16/14	1.35/0.83/3.2	N/A	12.9/26.4/9.7
Maranzano et al,[22] 2011	GBM	13/9	GKRS/HSRT	17/30 (10 fractions)	5.3/44	4	11
Conti et al,[20] 2012	GBM	12/11	CyberKnife (+/− temozolom ide)	20 (2 fractions)	13.1/18.4	66.7%/18% at 6 mo	12/7
Fogh et al,[18] 2010	GBM, AA	147	HSRT	35 (10 fractions)	22	N/A	11

Abbreviations: AA, anaplastic astrocytoma; AOA, anaplastic oligoastrocytoma; GBM, glioblastoma; GKRS, gamma knife radiosurgery; HSRT, hypofractionated stereotactic radiation therapy.
Data from Refs.[18–25]

bevacizumab use.[26–28] Reasons for this combination include sensitization of tumor endothelium to radiotherapy by vascular endothelial growth factor–depleting agents[29] and the potent antipermeability effect of bevacizumab potentially lessening the risk of radiation necrosis caused by SRS.[30] In the treatment of glioblastoma with hypofractionated stereotactic radiotherapy, the Sloan-Kettering group reported an objective radiographic response rate of 50% and a PFS rate at 6 months of 65% without radiation necrosis by combining radiotherapy with bevacizumab,[26] comparing favorably with outcomes in historical controls[31] or those in randomized trials of bevacizumab for recurrent glioblastoma.[15] Similarly, SRS has also been used concurrently with bevacizumab for recurrent high-grade glioma, and retrospective studies unanimously indicated potential benefit.[28,29] The Duke group compared outcomes of 42 patients with recurrent high-grade glioma treated with SRS combined with bevacizumab and those of 21 patients treated with SRS alone.[28] PFS and OS from SRS were better in patients treated with the combined therapy (median PFS 5.2 months vs 2.1 months, $P = .005$; median OS 11.2 months vs 3.9 months, $P = .014$, respectively). Similarly, a retrospective study by the Pittsburgh group reported improved patient survival from the time of SRS when survival of 11 patients with recurrent glioblastoma treated with SRS and bevacizumab was compared with that of 44 case-matched controls who underwent SRS without bevacizumab (median PFS 15 months vs 7 months, $P = .035$; median OS 18 months vs 12 months, $P = .005$, respectively).[27] A striking variation in patient survival between the above 2 retrospective studies may highlight their limitations; small numbers of accrued patients and potential selection bias would preclude definitive conclusions regarding the plausibility of the combined treatment. Two clinical trials are currently ongoing (NCT01086345, NCT01392209) to prospectively assess the efficacy and safety of SRS and concurrent bevacizumab in the treatment of recurrent high-grade glioma.

One potential flaw with SRS techniques in glioma treatment would be targeting the visible contrast enhancing lesion,[32] which may reflect a high rate of local recurrence.[33,34] Extended-field SRS enlarging a target tumor volume by additional 0.5–1 cm beyond the enhancing portion was reported to achieve superior tumor control to conventional SRS (93% vs 47%, $P = .035$) without increased rate of radiation necrosis.[35] Of note, the authors concluded that it failed to suppress remote dissemination sufficiently to enhance patient survival (**Fig. 1**). Given that an area of contrast enhancement on anatomic imaging does not necessarily coincide with an area of cell viability on metabolic imaging,[36] some groups have used magnetic resonance spectroscopy[37,38] or positron-emission tomography[39] to define more accurately areas of viable tumor.

RADIOSURGERY FOR LOW-GRADE GLIOMAS

SRS has also been applied to more benign, WHO grade I and II tumors, including diffuse astrocytoma and pilocytic astrocytoma. Those tumors are initially treated with as maximal surgical resection as possible, given the unequivocal association between gross total resection and enhanced patient survival.[40–42] Therefore, SRS is considered an option mainly for small residual tumors, tumors not amenable to resection such as deep-seated lesions and those in the eloquent brain, and recurrent tumors.[43]

The infiltrative nature of diffuse astrocytoma and oligodendroglioma warrants additional therapy to surgical resection in most cases, and fractionated radiotherapy is given at some point during the course of treatment, either right after the initial resection or at recurrence. The best evidence supports up-front radiotherapy, achieving a better PFS.[44] A caveat would be the lack of difference in OS; those who are concerned for up-front radiotherapy emphasize delayed cognitive dysfunction and impaired quality of life due to radiation effect.[45] In this regard, SRS may be just enough to control the tumor in carefully selected patients while sparing fractionated radiotherapy. There have been only small retrospective studies reported in the literature on SRS for diffuse astrocytoma.[43,46–48] Twenty-five patients with newly diagnosed or recurrent diffuse astrocytoma were treated with SRS at the University of Pittsburgh.[43] At a median follow-up of 65 months, tumor control was observed in half of the patients and the PFS rates after SRS were 91.3, 54.1, and 37.1% at 1, 5, and 10 years, respectively. For oligodendroglial tumors, the OS rates from diagnosis were 90.2% and 68.2% at 5 and 10 years, respectively.[49] These results suggest that SRS may be an active treatment of diffuse astrocytoma and oligodendroglioma. Prospective studies are warranted to assess the long-term efficacy and safety of SRS better for those low-grade gliomas.

SRS has been used either as a salvage therapy for recurrent ependymoma or as a boost to fractionated radiotherapy following surgical resection for newly diagnosed tumors. The paucity of chemotherapy options for ependymoma necessitates durable tumor control solely with radiation treatment. A retrospective study of 39 patients

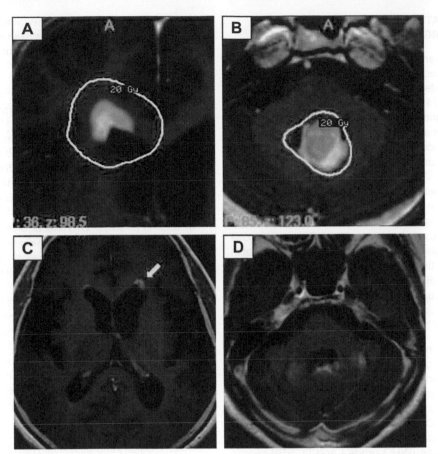

Fig. 1. Extended-field stereotactic radiosurgery (SRS) for recurrent glioblastoma. A 65-year-old woman diagnosed with left frontal glioblastoma underwent surgical resection followed by radiation therapy and temozolomide. (*A*) A new disseminated lesion was treated with extended-field SRS 7 months from diagnosis. (*B*) Two additional disseminated lesions including one in the fourth ventricle were treated with repeated SRS 3 months after the initial SRS. (*C, D*) Despite the durable tumor control for all the treated lesions after 2 months, several new lesions were found (*arrow*). The patient expired 2 months later, 14 months from diagnosis.

(56 tumors) treated at the University of Pittsburgh reported fair local control with PFS rates of 81.6, 45.8, and 45.8% at 1, 3, and 5 years after SRS, respectively.[50] All patients received SRS for recurrent tumors, except for 3 patients who underwent SRS for newly diagnosed tumors. Of note, histopathological grade was not associated with PFS among 34 WHO grade 2 tumors (25 patients) and 22 WHO grade 3 tumors (14 patients) in this series. The Mayo Clinic group reported actuarial tumor control rates of 85% and 72% at 1 and 3 years after SRS in their study of 26 recurrent ependymoma patients (49 tumors).[51] The propensity for dissemination apparently limits the durability of SRS treatment in ependymoma.[50,51]

Pilocytic astrocytoma, graded as WHO grade 1, can potentially be cured with complete removal; re-resection may be considered for residual tumors and recurrent tumors as long as they are surgically accessible with accepted risks. On the contrary, deep-seated lesions such as thalamic pilocytic astrocytoma may well be treated with SRS instead of surgical resection. The Pittsburgh group reported the largest retrospective studies in adult and pediatric populations.[52,53] The actuarial tumor control rates were 91.7, 82.8, and 70.8% at 1, 3, and 5 years from SRS, respectively, for 50 pediatric patients, and 83.9, 31.5, and 31.5%, respectively, for 14 adult patients. Delayed cyst progression seemed to hamper prolonged tumor control. The report from Mayo Clinic demonstrated similar tumor control rates: 65, 41, 15% at 1, 5, and 10 years after SRS.[54] Despite the histopathologically benign nature of pilocytic astrocytoma, it often does not behave benignly from clinical perspectives, especially in adults.[42,55] Indeed, long-term patient survival is often not seen, prompting additional management approaches besides SRS.[52]

COMPLICATIONS AFTER GLIOMA RADIOSURGERY

SRS is given to the irradiated brain, and thus, radiation necrosis is concerning as a late complication. Mehta and colleagues[10] reported 4 of 29 cases (14%) with brain necrosis in a series of newly diagnosed glioblastoma patients, and the prospective study of Kong and colleagues[19] noted radiation necrosis in 24% of patients (22 of 114 patients). In a prospective study by Chamberlain and colleagues,[56] 7 of 20 patients (35%) with recurrent glioblastoma developed early side effects (increased intracranial pressure) from SRS. All of them subsequently recovered without neurologic sequelae except one, who died. SRS may improve patient survival and achieve good tumor control in selected patients, but the risk of radiation necrosis is not insignificant. Therefore, SRS should only be offered to carefully selected patients.

SUMMARY

Despite numerous studies arguing for SRS for high-grade glioma, its efficacy does not seem totally convincing, warranting some refinement of this treatment. Preliminary results of recurrent glioblastoma treatment with SRS combined with bevacizumab are promising in terms of tumor response as well as patient survival. For low-grade gliomas (WHO grade I and II), SRS seems to achieve tumor response in many cases, but its long-term efficacy remains unclear given the favorable prognosis of the disease of many of these patients.

REFERENCES

1. Dolecek TA, Propp JM, Stroup NE, et al. CBTRUS statistical report: primary brain and central nervous system tumors diagnosed in the United States in 2005-2009. Neuro Oncol 2012;14(Suppl 5):v1–49.
2. Brandes AA, Tosoni A, Franceschi E, et al. Recurrence pattern after temozolomide concomitant with and adjuvant to radiotherapy in newly diagnosed patients with glioblastoma: correlation with MGMT promoter methylation status. J Clin Oncol 2009;27:1275–9.
3. Milano MT, Okunieff P, Donatello RS, et al. Patterns and timing of recurrence after temozolomide-based chemoradiation for glioblastoma. Int J Radiat Oncol Biol Phys 2010;78:1147–55.
4. Tanaka M, Ino Y, Nakagawa K, et al. High-dose conformal radiotherapy for supratentorial malignant glioma: a historical comparison. Lancet Oncol 2005;6:953–60.
5. Sarkaria JN, Mehta MP, Loeffler JS, et al. Radiosurgery in the initial management of malignant gliomas: survival comparison with the RTOG recursive partitioning analysis. Radiation Therapy Oncology Group. Int J Radiat Oncol Biol Phys 1995;32:931–41.
6. Nwokedi EC, DiBiase SJ, Jabbour S, et al. Gamma knife stereotactic radiosurgery for patients with glioblastoma multiforme. Neurosurgery 2002;50: 41–6 [discussion: 46–7].
7. Shrieve DC, Alexander E 3rd, Black PM, et al. Treatment of patients with primary glioblastoma multiforme with standard postoperative radiotherapy and radiosurgical boost: prognostic factors and long-term outcome. J Neurosurg 1999; 90:72–7.
8. Gannett D, Stea B, Lulu B, et al. Stereotactic radiosurgery as an adjunct to surgery and external beam radiotherapy in the treatment of patients with malignant gliomas. Int J Radiat Oncol Biol Phys 1995;33:461–8.
9. Loeffler JS, Alexander E 3rd, Shea WM, et al. Radiosurgery as part of the initial management of patients with malignant gliomas. J Clin Oncol 1992;10:1379–85.
10. Mehta MP, Masciopinto J, Rozental J, et al. Stereotactic radiosurgery for glioblastoma multiforme: report of a prospective study evaluating prognostic factors and analyzing long-term survival advantage. Int J Radiat Oncol Biol Phys 1994;30:541–9.
11. Shenouda G, Souhami L, Podgorsak EB, et al. Radiosurgery and accelerated radiotherapy for patients with glioblastoma. Can J Neurol Sci 1997;24: 110–5.
12. Tsao MN, Mehta MP, Whelan TJ, et al. The American Society for Therapeutic Radiology and Oncology (ASTRO) evidence-based review of the role of radiosurgery for malignant glioma. Int J Radiat Oncol Biol Phys 2005;63:47–55.
13. Souhami L, Seiferheld W, Brachman D, et al. Randomized comparison of stereotactic radiosurgery followed by conventional radiotherapy with carmustine to conventional radiotherapy with carmustine for patients with glioblastoma multiforme: report of Radiation Therapy Oncology Group 93-05 protocol. Int J Radiat Oncol Biol Phys 2004;60:853–60.
14. Lai A, Tran A, Nghiemphu PL, et al. Phase II study of bevacizumab plus temozolomide during and after radiation therapy for patients with newly diagnosed glioblastoma multiforme. J Clin Oncol 2011; 29:142–8.
15. Friedman HS, Prados MD, Wen PY, et al. Bevacizumab alone and in combination with irinotecan in recurrent glioblastoma. J Clin Oncol 2009;27: 4733–40.
16. Narayana A, Kunnakkat SD, Medabalmi P, et al. Change in pattern of relapse after antiangiogenic therapy in high-grade glioma. Int J Radiat Oncol Biol Phys 2012;82:77–82.

17. Norden AD, Young GS, Setayesh K, et al. Bevacizumab for recurrent malignant gliomas: efficacy, toxicity, and patterns of recurrence. Neurology 2008;70:779–87.

18. Fogh SE, Andrews DW, Glass J, et al. Hypofractionated stereotactic radiation therapy: an effective therapy for recurrent high-grade gliomas. J Clin Oncol 2010;28:3048–53.

19. Kong DS, Lee JI, Park K, et al. Efficacy of stereotactic radiosurgery as a salvage treatment for recurrent malignant gliomas. Cancer 2008;112:2046–51.

20. Conti A, Pontoriero A, Arpa D, et al. Efficacy and toxicity of CyberKnife re-irradiation and "dose dense" temozolomide for recurrent gliomas. Acta Neurochir (Wien) 2012;154:203–9.

21. Patel M, Siddiqui F, Jin JY, et al. Salvage reirradiation for recurrent glioblastoma with radiosurgery: radiographic response and improved survival. J Neurooncol 2009;92:185–91.

22. Maranzano E, Anselmo P, Casale M, et al. Treatment of recurrent glioblastoma with stereotactic radiotherapy: long-term results of a mono-institutional trial. Tumori 2011;97:56–61.

23. Pouratian N, Crowley RW, Sherman JH, et al. Gamma Knife radiosurgery after radiation therapy as an adjunctive treatment for glioblastoma. J Neurooncol 2009;94:409–18.

24. Elliott RE, Parker EC, Rush SC, et al. Efficacy of gamma knife radiosurgery for small-volume recurrent malignant gliomas after initial radical resection. World Neurosurg 2010;76:128–40 [discussion: 161–2].

25. Villavicencio AT, Burneikiene S, Romanelli P, et al. Survival following stereotactic radiosurgery for newly diagnosed and recurrent glioblastoma multiforme: a multicenter experience. Neurosurg Rev 2009;32(4):417–24.

26. Gutin PH, Iwamoto FM, Beal K, et al. Safety and efficacy of bevacizumab with hypofractionated stereotactic irradiation for recurrent malignant gliomas. Int J Radiat Oncol Biol Phys 2009;75:156–63.

27. Park KJ, Kano H, Iyer A, et al. Salvage gamma knife stereotactic radiosurgery followed by bevacizumab for recurrent glioblastoma multiforme: a case-control study. J Neurooncol 2012;107:323–33.

28. Cuneo KC, Vredenburgh JJ, Sampson JH, et al. Safety and efficacy of stereotactic radiosurgery and adjuvant bevacizumab in patients with recurrent malignant gliomas. Int J Radiat Oncol Biol Phys 2012;82:2018–24.

29. Gorski DH, Beckett MA, Jaskowiak NT, et al. Blockage of the vascular endothelial growth factor stress response increases the antitumor effects of ionizing radiation. Cancer Res 1999;59:3374–8.

30. Levin VA, Bidaut L, Hou P, et al. Randomized double-blind placebo-controlled trial of bevacizumab therapy for radiation necrosis of the central nervous system. Int J Radiat Oncol Biol Phys 2011;79:1487–95.

31. Wong ET, Hess KR, Gleason MJ, et al. Outcomes and prognostic factors in recurrent glioma patients enrolled onto phase II clinical trials. J Clin Oncol 1999;17:2572–8.

32. Sheehan J. Stereotactic radiosurgery for glioblastoma–time to revisit this approach. World Neurosurg 2012;78:592–3.

33. Shrieve DC, Alexander E 3rd, Wen PY, et al. Comparison of stereotactic radiosurgery and brachytherapy in the treatment of recurrent glioblastoma multiforme. Neurosurgery 1995;36:275–82 [discussion: 282–4].

34. Hall WA, Djalilian HR, Sperduto PW, et al. Stereotactic radiosurgery for recurrent malignant gliomas. J Clin Oncol 1995;13:1642–8.

35. Koga T, Maruyama K, Tanaka M, et al. Extended field stereotactic radiosurgery for recurrent glioblastoma. Cancer 2011;118:4193–200.

36. Miwa K, Shinoda J, Yano H, et al. Discrepancy between lesion distributions on methionine PET and MR images in patients with glioblastoma multiforme: insight from a PET and MR fusion image study. J Neurol Neurosurg Psychiatry 2004;75:1457–62.

37. Einstein DB, Wessels B, Bangert B, et al. Phase II trial of radiosurgery to magnetic resonance spectroscopy-defined high-risk tumor volumes in patients with glioblastoma multiforme. Int J Radiat Oncol Biol Phys 2012;84:668–74.

38. Graves EE, Nelson SJ, Vigneron DB, et al. A preliminary study of the prognostic value of proton magnetic resonance spectroscopic imaging in gamma knife radiosurgery of recurrent malignant gliomas. Neurosurgery 2000;46:319–26 [discussion: 326–8].

39. Grosu AL, Weber WA, Franz M, et al. Reirradiation of recurrent high-grade gliomas using amino acid PET (SPECT)/CT/MRI image fusion to determine gross tumor volume for stereotactic fractionated radiotherapy. Int J Radiat Oncol Biol Phys 2005;63:511–9.

40. McGirt MJ, Chaichana KL, Attenello FJ, et al. Extent of surgical resection is independently associated with survival in patients with hemispheric infiltrating low-grade gliomas. Neurosurgery 2008;63:700–7 [author reply: 707–8].

41. Smith JS, Chang EF, Lamborn KR, et al. Role of extent of resection in the long-term outcome of low-grade hemispheric gliomas. J Clin Oncol 2008;26:1338–45.

42. Stuer C, Vilz B, Majores M, et al. Frequent recurrence and progression in pilocytic astrocytoma in adults. Cancer 2007;110:2799–808.

43. Park KJ, Kano H, Kondziolka D, et al. Early or delayed radiosurgery for WHO grade II astrocytomas. J Neurooncol 2011;103:523–32.

44. van den Bent MJ, Afra D, de Witte O, et al. Long-term efficacy of early versus delayed radiotherapy for low-grade astrocytoma and oligodendroglioma in adults: the EORTC 22845 randomised trial. Lancet 2005;366:985–90.

45. Kiebert GM, Curran D, Aaronson NK, et al. Quality of life after radiation therapy of cerebral low-grade gliomas of the adult: results of a randomised phase III trial on dose response (EORTC trial 22844). EORTC Radiotherapy Co-operative Group. Eur J Cancer 1998;34:1902–9.

46. Hadjipanayis CG, Niranjan A, Tyler-Kabara E, et al. Stereotactic radiosurgery for well-circumscribed fibrillary grade II astrocytomas: an initial experience. Stereotact Funct Neurosurg 2002;79:13–24.

47. Kida Y, Kobayashi T, Mori Y. Gamma knife radiosurgery for low-grade astrocytomas: results of long-term follow up. J Neurosurg 2000;93(Suppl 3):42–6.

48. Wang LW, Shiau CY, Chung WY, et al. Gamma Knife surgery for low-grade astrocytomas: evaluation of long-term outcome based on a 10-year experience. J Neurosurg 2006;105(Suppl):127–32.

49. Kano H, Niranjan A, Khan A, et al. Does radiosurgery have a role in the management of oligodendrogliomas? J Neurosurg 2009;110:564–71.

50. Kano H, Niranjan A, Kondziolka D, et al. Outcome predictors for intracranial ependymoma radiosurgery. Neurosurgery 2009;64:279–87 [discussion: 287–8].

51. Stauder MC, Ni Laack N, Ahmed KA, et al. Stereotactic radiosurgery for patients with recurrent intracranial ependymomas. J Neurooncol 2012;108: 507–12.

52. Kano H, Kondziolka D, Niranjan A, et al. Stereotactic radiosurgery for pilocytic astrocytomas part 1: outcomes in adult patients. J Neurooncol 2009; 95:211–8.

53. Kano H, Niranjan A, Kondziolka D, et al. Stereotactic radiosurgery for pilocytic astrocytomas part 2: outcomes in pediatric patients. J Neurooncol 2009;95:219–29.

54. Hallemeier CL, Pollock BE, Schomberg PJ, et al. Stereotactic radiosurgery for recurrent or unresectable pilocytic astrocytoma. Int J Radiat Oncol Biol Phys 2012;83:107–12.

55. Johnson DR, Brown PD, Galanis E, et al. Pilocytic astrocytoma survival in adults: analysis of the Surveillance, Epidemiology, and End Results Program of the National Cancer Institute. J Neurooncol 2012;108:187–93.

56. Chamberlain MC, Barba D, Kormanik P, et al. Stereotactic radiosurgery for recurrent gliomas. Cancer 1994;74:1342–7.

Radiosurgical Management of Trigeminal Neuralgia

Michael D. Chan, MD[a],*, Edward G. Shaw, MD, MA[a],
Stephen B. Tatter, MD, PhD[b]

KEYWORDS

- Trigeminal neuralgia • Stereotactic radiosurgery • Facial pain

KEY POINTS

- Stereotactic radiosurgery represents a safe and effective noninvasive treatment option for patients with trigeminal neuralgia.
- The major limitation of radiosurgery as compared with microvascular decompression is the limited durability of pain relief.
- Optimal populations for radiosurgery include patients older than 70 years, patients with multiple sclerosis, and patients with significant medical comorbidities.

INTRODUCTION

Trigeminal neuralgia, also known as *tic douloureux*, is a severe paroxysmal facial pain located within the trigeminal distribution on the face. This condition has been described as a "suicide disease" because of the severe intensity of the pain. Approximately 45 000 people in the United States have been diagnosed with trigeminal neuralgia.

Classification and Cause

Trigeminal neuralgia is one of several different types of facial pain that can have similar characteristics. The most widely accepted classification scheme for facial pain was published by Burchiel.[1] The Burchiel classification is summarized in **Table 1**. Classic idiopathic trigeminal neuralgia is known as type I trigeminal neuralgia in the Burchiel classification. It is defined as pain that is episodic at least 50% of the time. It is located within any of the 3 divisions of the trigeminal nerve. It is also commonly described as sharp, stabbing, or electrical shocklike in quality. The intensity of the pain

has been described using the Barrow Neurologic Institute (BNI) pain scale. This scale is commonly used in the scientific literature to describe pain before and after an intervention and to compare results between multiple series. The BNI scale is summarized in **Table 2**.

The pathophysiology of type I trigeminal neuralgia has been explained by what has become known as the *vascular hypothesis*. This hypothesis posits that the episodic pain syndrome of trigeminal neuralgia is caused by compression of the trigeminal nerve by a blood vessel.[2] The most common offending vessel is the superior cerebellar artery. It is also thought that the brain settles within the cranial vault with age and, thus, creates a greater likelihood for such an interaction between blood vessel and trigeminal nerve in the more elderly population.

Other causes that can produce pain syndromes similar to idiopathic trigeminal neuralgia include multiple sclerosis, tumors of the skull base (eg, meningioma, acoustic neuroma, metastatic disease), Charcot-Marie-Tooth disease, Lyme disease, herpes zoster, traumatic nerve injury, and

Disclosures: The authors have nothing to disclose.
[a] Department of Radiation Oncology, Wake Forest School of Medicine, Medical Center Boulevard, Winston-Salem, NC 27157, USA; [b] Department of Neurosurgery, Wake Forest School of Medicine, Medical Center Boulevard, Winston-Salem, NC 27157, USA
* Corresponding author.
E-mail address: mchan@wakehealth.edu

Neurosurg Clin N Am 24 (2013) 613–621
http://dx.doi.org/10.1016/j.nec.2013.05.001
1042-3680/13/$ – see front matter © 2013 Elsevier Inc. All rights reserved.

Table 1
Burchiel classification scheme for facial pain

Diagnosis	Clinical History
Type I trigeminal neuralgia	>50% episodic pain
Type II trigeminal neuralgia	<50% episodic pain
Trigeminal neuropathic pain	Caused by unintentional trauma (eg, tooth extraction)
Trigeminal deafferentation pain	Caused by intentional trauma (eg, rhizotomy)
Symptomatic trigeminal neuralgia	Multiple sclerosis
Postherpetic neuralgia	Herpes zoster outbreak in trigeminal distribution
Atypical facial pain	Somatoform pain

somatoform pain disorders. The importance of the various causes of facial pain with regard to the use of stereotactic radiosurgery (SRS) is the fact that radiosurgical management has a high rate of response for type I pain but an inferior response rate for some of the other causes. The risk of SRS-related toxicity, although low, is another reason to differentiate between the various causes of facial pain. Patients with herpetic neuralgia and neuropathic pain from traumatic nerve injury are unlikely to respond to radiosurgery.

THERAPEUTIC OPTIONS

Several treatment options have evolved over time, including the use of antiepileptic medications, microvascular decompression (MVD) surgery, percutaneous rhizotomy, and SRS. The treatment option used for each individual case depends on

Table 2
BNI pain intensity scale

Pain Score	Definition
I	No trigeminal pain, no medication
II	Occasional pain, not requiring medication
III	Some pain, adequately controlled with medication
IV	Some pain, not adequately controlled with medication
V	Severe pain, no pain relief

factors such as patients' age, medical comorbidities, and prior treatment options that have either succeeded or failed. A proposed management algorithm is depicted in **Fig. 1**.

Medical Management

The first-line therapeutic option for newly diagnosed trigeminal neuralgia is medical management. In general, antiepileptics are the most common type of medication used for trigeminal neuralgia, though tricyclic antidepressants, benzodiazepines, and narcotics have all been used. The single most effective medication for trigeminal neuralgia is carbamazepine (Tegretol). Other medications that have reported responses include phenytoin (Dilantin), baclofen (Gablofen), oxcarbazepine (Trileptal), gabapentin (Neurontin), and lamotrigine (Lamictal). Patients who have an initial response to medical management can undergo a trial of withdrawal of medications over time as the pain may undergo remission. It is not uncommon, however, for patients to become refractory to medical management over time, and these patients will commonly require surgical or ablative management. Furthermore, some of the antiepileptics will commonly have associated toxicities, such as sedation, cognitive changes, and ataxia. Carbamazepine, in particular, can have a high rate of such toxicities. Oxcarbazepine and gabapentin may have lower rates of toxicity. A common indication for surgical or radiosurgical intervention is when patients experience medication-related toxicity from antiepileptics that start to affect their quality of life.

MVD

MVD is a surgical technique involving a craniotomy and decompression of the trigeminal nerve from the offending blood vessel. Intraoperative insertion of an inert implant (generally Teflon, DuPont, Wilmington, DE) allows for the prevention of recurrent vascular compression. The chief advantage of MVD is the fact that the pain relief is durable and likely curative. In general, 70% of patients treated with MVD continue to be pain free 20 years after the operation.[3] Operative morbidity and mortality is generally quite low but increases after 70 years of age, which is the age that noninvasive alternatives may have a greater therapeutic ratio.[4]

SRS

SRS represents a noninvasive treatment option for trigeminal neuralgia, with its main advantage being its noninvasiveness and low morbidity rate. Most of the data that exist for radiosurgical management of trigeminal neuralgia is using the Gamma Knife

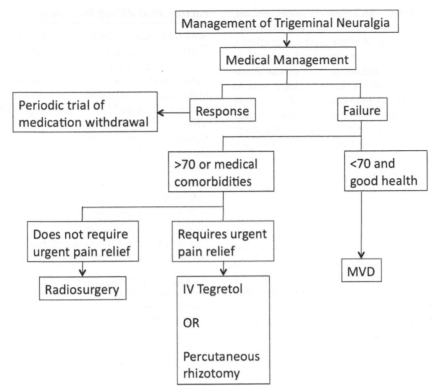

Fig. 1. Management algorithm for trigeminal neuralgia.

(Elekta, Stockholm, Sweden), although there is an emerging literature for linear accelerator approaches. The major disadvantage of SRS is the limitation in the durability of the pain response. Most series have shown that the median duration of radiosurgical response to be on the order of 5 years. Although SRS can be repeated, for younger patients, even a second application of SRS may not remain effective throughout their lifespan. Elderly patients and those with surgical contraindications, such as severe cerebrovascular or cardiovascular disease or bleeding diatheses, may also be best treated with a radiosurgical approach.

Percutaneous Rhizotomy

Percutaneous ablative techniques have also shown success in the treatment of trigeminal neuralgia. These techniques include radiofrequency rhizotomy, glycerol rhizotomy, and balloon rhizotomy. The chief advantage of percutaneous ablative techniques is that pain relief is immediate and that they often do not require general anesthesia. Comparison of the percutaneous procedures has suggested that they likely have very similar response rates and durability of response. However, the likelihood of persistent hypesthesia may be higher than what is seen with MVD or a

radiosurgical approach. The durability of response for percutaneous techniques is limited and similar to results with SRS.

OUTCOMES AFTER TRIGEMINAL NEURALGIA RADIOSURGERY

Because most of the data for radiosurgical outcomes have come using the Gamma Knife unit, for the purpose of this review, the following radiosurgical outcomes will refer specifically to Gamma Knife radiosurgery (GKRS) results, with the exception of the section specifically dedicated to linear accelerator approaches.

Prospective Studies

There are few prospective studies for the use of SRS in the treatment of trigeminal neuralgia.[5–7] The first such study was a prospective study performed by a group from Marseille, France and was a quality-of-life assessment showing improvement in all quality-of-life parameters and finding that 58 of 83 (70%) responders were able to come off of medications.[5] A second prospective study conducted at the Mayo Clinic looked at the cost-effectiveness of SRS versus MVD as a definitive treatment option for trigeminal neuralgia.[6] In this study, MVD was more expensive in the near term; but for patients with longer life expectancies, it seemed to be the more cost-effective treatment option. The University of Pittsburgh conducted a randomized prospective study of 87 patients in which patients were randomized to 1 versus 2 isocenters.[7] The rationale for such a study was to determine whether an increased length of nerve treated resulted in any difference in either efficacy or toxicity of radiosurgical treatment. Although there was no change detected in efficacy, the incidence of complications correlated with the nerve length irradiated (more facial numbness with 2 isocenters vs 1 isocenter).

Response Rate and Durability of Pain Response

Several large retrospective series have also been reported for trigeminal neuralgia after definitive SRS.[8–18] The results of the largest series of GKRS for the treatment of trigeminal neuralgia are summarized in **Table 3**. The series that have been reported have been shown quite similar results regarding pain response. In a series from Wake Forest, Marshall and colleagues[14] reported a cohort of more than 400 patients with trigeminal neuralgia and reported an 86% initial response to pain within 3 months.

Among the greater concerns for treatment with SRS is the increasing possibility of pain relapse with increasing time after treatment. Riesenburger and colleagues[17] reported that pain relapse after SRS is a time-dependent phenomenon. Marshall and colleagues[14] reported a median durability of 4.9 years for patients with type I trigeminal neuralgia. Lucas and colleagues[12] have recently reported that the initial successful response and ability to discontinue medications was the dominant factor predicting durable pain relief after SRS.

Factors that Affect Response

Several factors have been identified that affect the likelihood of treatment success for SRS in the treatment of trigeminal neuralgia. The development of posttreatment numbness has been identified as a major factor that predicts the success of treatment in multiple series.[11,14,16] Prior surgery for trigeminal neuralgia[13] and particularly radiofrequency ablation of the nerve[14] seems to decrease the likelihood of treatment response. Regis and colleagues[5] showed a sequential decrease in response with every previous procedure performed. Having magnetic resonance imaging (MRI) evidence of contact between a blood vessel and the trigeminal nerve seems to predict a better response after SRS.[19] The dose rate of the Gamma Knife sources does not seem to affect the response rate.[20]

Radiosurgical Dosing

Doses delivered for SRS generally range between 70 and 90 Gy prescribed to the isocenter. There has been one series whereby patients were treated in the repeat setting and pain responses were seen at doses as low as 45 Gy prescribed to the isocenter.[21] Pollock and colleagues[22] reported results from the Mayo Clinic in which patients were treated with either 70 or 90 Gy. Patients in the 90-Gy cohort experienced a greater degree of pain relief but also had a greater degree of numbness. The mechanism of pain relief is thought to be focal axonal degeneration of the trigeminal nerve that affects pain fibers proportionately more than sensory fibers.[10] At higher doses, necrosis is seen more commonly and may contribute to the response to SRS.[23] The upper limit of the acceptable dose range seems to be 90 Gy because several large publications have used this dose and found it to be safe.[5,15,24]

Table 3
Selected large series of Gamma Knife radiosurgery for trigeminal neuralgia

Institution	Number	Median Dose (Gy)	Response Rate (%)	Any Toxicity (%)
Pittsburgh	503	80	89	11
Marseille	497	85	91	14
Wake Forest	448	90	86	44
Columbia	293	75	76	5
University of Virginia	136	80	90	19
Mayo	117	90	85	37
Maryland	112	75	81	6[a]
Brussels	109	90	82	38[b]

[a] Series reported bothersome numbness only.
[b] Beam channel blocking was used in this series.
Data from Refs.[5,8,10,14,16–18,38]

Type II Trigeminal Neuralgia

Several reports have demonstrated a decreased response rate and durability of response in patients with type II trigeminal neuralgia when treated with surgical or radiosurgical modalities. Tyler-Kabara and colleagues[25] showed that, in series of 2264 patients with trigeminal neuralgia, those with type II pain had a greater risk of relapsing over time as compared with patients with type I pain. There have been much more limited series assessing the outcomes of patients with non–type I trigeminal neuralgia after SRS. This population has been difficult to assess because of the heterogeneity of the population in general and the nonstandardized classification systems used by various institutions. Dhople and colleagues[9] published a series of 35 patients with atypical trigeminal neuralgia from the University of Maryland. In this series, the investigators encompassed patients with type II pain (continuous) as well as patients with burning as opposed to lancinating pain. There was a trend toward longer time before pain relief and shorter duration of pain relief in patients with atypical trigeminal neuralgia in this series.

A series from Wake Forest University compared outcomes of patients with type I and type II trigeminal neuralgia.[14] In this series, there were 61 patients with type II trigeminal neuralgia and 32 patients with atypical facial pain. Patients with type II trigeminal neuralgia and atypical facial pain both had decreased initial response rates after SRS as well as a decreased durability of pain relief. Median durability of pain relief was 4.9 years for type I, 1.7 years for type II, and 0.7 years for atypical facial pain.

MS-Related Trigeminal Neuralgia

Multiple sclerosis (MS)-related, also called *symptomatic*, trigeminal neuralgia comprises approximately 1% of patients with trigeminal neuralgialike symptoms. The most important distinction in this population with regard to therapeutic options is the difference in pathophysiology of the pain. MS-related trigeminal neuralgia is caused by a demyelinating process within the trigeminal neuronal pathway. Microvascular decompression is not considered an adequate treatment option because it does not address the pathophysiology of the disease. Medical management is considered to be the first-line therapy like it is for idiopathic trigeminal neuralgia. Surgical options, such as glycerol rhizotomy and SRS, have also been reported. Because of the relative rarity of symptomatic trigeminal neuralgia, available published evidence is limited to small single-institution retrospective series. In one such study published by the University of Pittsburgh, 37 patients were treated with GKRS using a dose range between 70 and 90 Gy.[26] The investigators reported that 36 of 37 patients reported BNI I-IIIb pain at some point in their course, with 23 patients experiencing a BNI I pain score. Five percent of patients experienced a new-onset paresthesia in this series.

Bilateral Trigeminal Neuralgia

Bilateral trigeminal neuralgia is a complicated clinical entity that represents approximately 2% of patients with trigeminal neuralgia. The cause of bilateral trigeminal neuralgia is commonly related to either Charcot-Marie-Tooth disease or multiple sclerosis.[27] It has been shown that patients with bilateral trigeminal neuralgia are less likely to have blood vessel compression on MRI[19] and, thus, likely that a proportion of these patients have pain that is not caused by vascular compression. The clinical complexity of the bilateral pain is related to the possibility of bilateral trigeminal nerve dysfunction that can result from an ablative treatment. The efficacy of MVD is in question given the difference in pathophysiology of the patients with bilateral pain. SRS for bilateral trigeminal neuralgia has been reported in an 8-patient series by Tufts Medical Center without significant toxicity.[28] However, long-term efficacy remains to be reported. One approach to avoid bilateral trigeminal nerve dysfunction has been to treat the more symptomatic side first, then follow patients for 6 to 12 months to assess for efficacy and toxicity before deciding on the management of the other side.

Repeat Radiosurgery

Because the median durability of pain relief after SRS is on the order of 5 years, more than half of patients receiving primary SRS will have a recurrence of trigeminal neuralgia pain at some point in their lifetime. In this scenario, a second application of SRS is a reasonable treatment option. Several institutions have now reported on the efficacy of repeat SRS and found that the response rate and durability of a second response are similar to what is seen with the first application.[21,29–35] Select results of repeat radiosurgical series are presented in **Table 4**.

Patient selection is an important issue in patients who are considered for a second radiosurgical procedure. A detailed history is necessary to rule out the possibility that the pain patients are experiencing is truly a recurrence of trigeminal neuralgia as opposed to a consequence of previous SRS, such as deafferentation pain. A common

Table 4
Repeat radiosurgery series for relapsed trigeminal neuralgia

Institution	Number	Median Retreatment Dose (Gy)	Response Rate (%)	Any Toxicity (%)
Mayo	19	76	95	21
Columbia	45	40	62	13
Wake Forest	37	84	84	57
Tufts	27	45	86	29
Medical University of Graz	22	74	100	74
Pittsburgh	119	70	87	21
Maryland	18	70	78	11
Tangdu Hospital (China)	34	71	97	12

Data from Refs.[21,29–35]

practice is to select patients who had a good pain outcome after their initial SRS.

Linear Accelerator-Based Approaches

Linear accelerator-based approaches for trigeminal neuralgia are used less than Gamma Knife SRS for several reasons, including the difficulty in accurately characterizing the output factor for a 4-mm collimator, the instability associated with a linear accelerator gantry, and the fact that inaccuracies are cumulative. The potential inaccuracy for a linear accelerator treatment of trigeminal neuralgia has been estimated to be as great as 30%. For sufficient treatment of trigeminal neuralgia on a linear accelerator using a 4-mm collimator, a root mean square value of all errors likely needs to be less than 1 mm.[36]

The largest series of linear accelerator-based SRS was published by a group from the University of California, Los Angeles.[24] In this series of 179 patients, the investigators demonstrated a response rate and durability of treatment similar to that seen with Gamma Knife series. A median dose of 90 Gy (range, 70–90 Gy) with the 30% isodose line tangential to the pons was used in this series.

RADIOSURGICAL TARGETING FOR TRIGEMINAL NEURALGIA

The technical goal of trigeminal neuralgia SRS is to place a radiosurgical 4-mm isocenter onto the trigeminal nerve as it runs through the prepontine cistern. The rationale for placing the isocenter within the prepontine cistern is that the nerve can be well visualized on MRI in this area and that the nerve is also surrounded by cerebrospinal fluid, allowing for the precise targeting and sharp dose falloff beyond the nerve, minimizing the risk

of damage to surrounding structures, such as the brainstem and temporal lobe.

There are several hypotheses on the target of radiation effect when trigeminal neuralgia is treated with SRS. The putative target of radiation damage is important because of the implications it has on the ideal isocenter location. Kondziolka and colleagues[10] have published that the dorsal root entry zone is more radiosensitive than more distal portions of the nerve because of the transition between more radiosensitive oligodendrocytes and more resistant Schwann cells. This finding was supported from data from Columbia University, which demonstrated improved pain outcomes in patients with greater volumes of brainstem receiving a dose of 15 Gy.[37] A strategy for targeting the dorsal root entry zone places the isocenter such that the 50% isodose line is tangential to the brainstem. However, data from multiple other series have reported equivalent pain relief while targeting a more distal portion of the nerve, such as the pars triangularis.[5]

Current targeting strategies include targeting the pars triangularis and using the 20% isodose line to determine the isocenter location (**Fig. 2**). The rationale for targeting the pars triangularis is that it is a relatively distal portion of the nerve but would allow targeting of the entire nerve circumference before it diverges into multiple branches. Other series have placed the 20% isodose line such that it is tangential to the brainstem surface. The rationale for this approach is to constrain the brainstem surface to less than 20 Gy because this dose has been implicated in treatment-related numbness. With this approach, it is common that most of the high-dose region is within the pars triangularis.

Another controversy regarding the targeting and delivery of SRS for trigeminal neuralgia involves

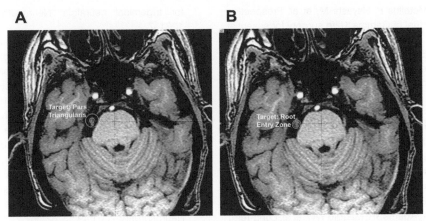

Fig. 2. Targeting strategies for trigeminal neuralgia radiosurgery. (*A*) Gamma Knife plan in which the target is the pars triangularis. In this plan, the 20% isodose line is tangential to the brain stem. (*B*) Gamma Knife plan in which the target is the dorsal root entry zone. In this plan, the 50% isodose line is tangential to the brainstem.

the question of collimator plugging. Plugging blocks a portion of the collimator to shape the beam to incorporate a greater length of nerve and to decrease the amount of brainstem exposure. A study from Brussels showed that the addition of plugging, although it modestly improved the response to the Gamma Knife, caused a greater degree of bothersome numbness.[38] The investigators concluded that plugging should be avoided.

There exists a population of patients with trigeminal neuralgia who are candidates for radiosurgical management but have contraindications to MRI, such as pacemaker placement, ferromagnetic implant, or shrapnel exposure. In such patients, computed tomography–based treatment planning has been reported in which the targeting of the nerve is done based on anatomic landmarks, such as the trigeminal impression on the temporal bone.[39,40] Further follow-up is likely necessary to ensure that this population does not have a higher rate of late toxicity or late pain recurrence.

RADIOSURGICAL COMPLICATIONS

Trigeminal nerve dysfunction is the major possible toxicity in patients who have received SRS for trigeminal neuralgia. The mechanism for such radiosurgical toxicity is damage to the sensory fibers within the trigeminal nerve. There have been several series that have reported higher rates of numbness in patients who have received higher doses and those who have a greater length of nerve treated. There has also been an association between patients who experience postradiosurgical numbness and the durability of radiosurgical treatment response.[11,14,16] Other series have suggested that excellent pain relief responses can be

achieved in the absence of trigeminal nerve dysfunction.[5,15] Recent data from the University of Pittsburgh suggest that patients receiving gabapentin may have a lesser risk of GKRS-induced numbness.[41] More severe toxicities that occur following SRS include corneal anesthesia and anesthesia dolorosa. The likelihood of more severe toxicity is rare, with anesthesia dolorosa rates reported to be less than 1%.

SUMMARY

SRS represents a safe and effective noninvasive treatment option for trigeminal neuralgia. The major limitation of SRS lies in its limited durability as compared with MVD. Patients older than 70 years with multiple sclerosis or significant medical comorbidities represent populations that may be best suited for SRS. Patients are generally best managed by a multidisciplinary team to determine which treatment option is optimal for each patient.

REFERENCES

1. Burchiel KJ. A new classification for facial pain. Neurosurgery 2003;53:1164–6.
2. Jannetta PJ. Arterial compression of the trigeminal nerve at the pons in patients with trigeminal neuralgia. J Neurosurg 1967;26:159–62.
3. Barker FG 2nd, Jannetta PJ, Bissonette DJ, et al. The long-term outcome of microvascular decompression for trigeminal neuralgia. N Engl J Med 1996;334:1077–83.
4. Kalkanis SN, Eskandar EN, Carter BS, et al. Microvascular decompression surgery in the United States, 1996 to 2000: mortality rates, morbidity rates, and the effects of hospital and surgeon volumes. Neurosurgery 2003;52:1251–62.

5. Regis J, Metellus P, Hayashi M, et al. Prospective controlled trial of Gamma Knife surgery for essential trigeminal neuralgia. J Neurosurg 2006;104:913–24.

6. Pollock BE, Ecker RD. A prospective cost-effectiveness study of trigeminal neuralgia surgery. Clin J Pain 2005;21:317–22.

7. Flickinger JC, Pollock BE, Kondziolka D, et al. Does increased nerve length within the treatment volume improve trigeminal neuralgia radiosurgery? A prospective double-blind, randomized study. Int J Radiat Oncol Biol Phys 2001;51:449–54.

8. Brisman R. Gamma Knife surgery with a dose of 75 to 76.8 Gray for trigeminal neuralgia. J Neurosurg 2004;100:848–54.

9. Dhople AA, Adams JR, Maggio WW, et al. Long-term outcomes of Gamma Knife radiosurgery for classic trigeminal neuralgia: implications of treatment and critical review of the literature. Clinical article. J Neurosurg 2009;111:351–8.

10. Kondziolka D, Lunsford LD, Flickinger JC, et al. Stereotactic radiosurgery for trigeminal neuralgia: a multiinstitutional study using the gamma unit. J Neurosurg 1996;84:940–5.

11. Kondziolka D, Zorro O, Lobato-Polo J, et al. Gamma Knife stereotactic radiosurgery for idiopathic trigeminal neuralgia. J Neurosurg 2010;112:758–65.

12. Lucas JT, Marshall K, Bourland JD, et al. Predictors of durability of response for stereotactic radiosurgery in the treatment of trigeminal neuralgia. Int J Radiat Oncol Biol Phys 2012;84:S37–8.

13. Maesawa S, Salame C, Flickinger JC, et al. Clinical outcomes after stereotactic radiosurgery for idiopathic trigeminal neuralgia. J Neurosurg 2001;94:14–20.

14. Marshall K, Chan MD, McCoy TP, et al. Predictive variables for the successful treatment of trigeminal neuralgia with gamma knife radiosurgery. Neurosurgery 2012;70:566–73.

15. Massager N, Lorenzoni J, Devriendt D, et al. Gamma knife surgery for idiopathic trigeminal neuralgia performed using a far-anterior cisternal target and a high dose of radiation. J Neurosurg 2004;100:597–605.

16. Pollock BE, Phuong LK, Gorman DA, et al. Stereotactic radiosurgery for idiopathic trigeminal neuralgia. J Neurosurg 2002;97:347–53.

17. Riesenburger RI, Hwang SW, Schirmer CM, et al. Outcomes following single treatment Gamma Knife surgery for trigeminal neuralgia with a minimum 3-year follow-up. J Neurosurg 2010;112:766–71.

18. Sheehan J, Pan HC, Stroila M, et al. Gamma Knife surgery for trigeminal neuralgia: outcomes and prognostic factors. J Neurosurg 2005;102:434–41.

19. Brisman R, Khandji AG, Mooij RB. Trigeminal nerve-blood vessel relationship as revealed by high-resolution magnetic resonance imaging and its effect on pain relief after Gamma Knife radiosurgery for trigeminal neuralgia. Neurosurgery 2002;50:1261–7.

20. Balamucki CJ, Stieber VW, Ellis TL, et al. Does dose rate affect efficacy? The outcomes of 256 gamma knife surgery procedures for trigeminal neuralgia and other types of facial pain as they relate to the half-life of cobalt. J Neurosurg 2006;105:730–5.

21. Dvorak T, Finn A, Price LL, et al. Retreatment of trigeminal neuralgia with Gamma Knife radiosurgery: is there an appropriate cumulative dose? Clinical article. J Neurosurg 2009;111:359–64.

22. Pollock BE, Phuong LK, Foote RL, et al. High-dose trigeminal neuralgia radiosurgery associated with increased risk of trigeminal nerve dysfunction. Neurosurgery 2001;49:58–62.

23. Kondziolka D, Lacomis D, Niranjan A, et al. Histological effects of trigeminal nerve radiosurgery in a primate model: implications for trigeminal neuralgia radiosurgery. Neurosurgery 2000;46:971–7.

24. Smith ZA, Gorgulho AA, Bezrukiy N, et al. Dedicated linear accelerator radiosurgery for trigeminal neuralgia: a single-center experience in 179 patients with varied dose prescriptions and treatment plans. Int J Radiat Oncol Biol Phys 2011;81:225–31.

25. Tyler-Kabara EC, Kassam AB, Horowitz MH, et al. Predictors of outcome in surgically managed patients with typical and atypical trigeminal neuralgia: comparison of results following microvascular decompression. J Neurosurg 2002;96:527–31.

26. Zorro O, Lobato-Polo J, Kano H, et al. Gamma Knife radiosurgery for multiple sclerosis-related trigeminal neuralgia. Neurology 2009;73:1149–54.

27. Tacconi L, Miles JB. Bilateral trigeminal neuralgia: a therapeutic dilemma. Br J Neurosurg 2000;14:33–9.

28. Wu JK, Raval A, Salluzzo J, et al. Results of bilateral trigeminal neuralgia treated with Gamma Knife radiosurgery: Boston Gamma Knife Center experience. Proceedings of 16th Meeting of the Leksell Gamma Knife Society, Sydney, March 25, 2012.

29. Aubuchon AC, Chan MD, Lovato JF, et al. Repeat Gamma Knife Radiosurgery for trigeminal neuralgia. Int J Radiat Oncol Biol Phys 2011;81:1059–65.

30. Brisman R. Repeat Gamma Knife radiosurgery for trigeminal neuralgia. Stereotact Funct Neurosurg 2003;81:43–9.

31. Gellner V, Kurschel S, Kreil W, et al. Recurrent trigeminal neuralgia: long-term outcome of repeat Gamma Knife radiosurgery. J Neurol Neurosurg Psychiatr 2008;79:1405–7.

32. Herman JM, Petit JH, Amin P, et al. Repeat Gamma Knife radiosurgery for refractory or recurrent trigeminal neuralgia: treatment outcomes and quality-of-life assessment. Int J Radiat Oncol Biol Phys 2004;59:112–6.

33. Park KJ, Kondziolka D, Berkowitz O, et al. Repeat Gamma Knife radiosurgery for trigeminal neuralgia. Neurosurgery 2012;70:295–305.

34. Pollock BE, Foote RL, Link MJ, et al. Repeat radio-surgery for idiopathic trigeminal neuralgia. Int J Radiat Oncol Biol Phys 2005;61:192–5.

35. Wang L, Zhao ZW, Qin HZ, et al. Repeat Gamma Knife radiosurgery for recurrent or refractory trigeminal neuralgia. Neurol India 2008;56:36–41.

36. Rahimian J, Chen JC, Rao AA, et al. Geometrical accuracy of the Novalis stereotactic radiosurgery system for trigeminal neuralgia. J Neurosurg 2004; 101(Suppl 3):351–5.

37. Brisman R, Mooij R. Gamma Knife radiosurgery for trigeminal neuralgia: dose-volume histograms of the brainstem and trigeminal nerve. J Neurosurg 2000;93(Suppl 3):155–8.

38. Massager N, Nissim O, Murata N, et al. Effect of beam channel plugging on the outcome of Gamma Knife radiosurgery for trigeminal neuralgia. Int J Radiat Oncol Biol Phys 2006;65:1200–5.

39. Attia A, Tatter SB, Weller M, et al. CT-only planning for Gamma Knife radiosurgery in the treatment of trigeminal neuralgia: methodology and outcomes from a single institution. J Med Imaging Radiat Oncol 2012;56:490–4.

40. Park KJ, Kano H, Berkowitz O, et al. Computed tomography-guided Gamma Knife stereotactic radiosurgery for trigeminal neuralgia. Acta Neurochir (Wien) 2011;153:1601–9.

41. Flickinger JC Jr, Kim H, Kano H, et al. Do carbamazepine, gabapentin, or other anticonvulsants exert sufficient radioprotective effects to alter responses from trigeminal neuralgia radiosurgery? Int J Radiat Oncol Biol Phys 2013;83:e501.

Stereotactic Radiosurgery for Epilepsy and Functional Disorders

Douglas Kondziolka, MD, MSc, FRCSC, FACS[a],*,
John C. Flickinger, MD, FACR[b], L. Dade Lunsford, MD, FACS[c]

KEYWORDS

- Stereotactic radiosurgery • Epilepsy • Gamma knife • Radiosurgical thalamotomy
- Radiosurgical pallidotomy • Pain • Behavioral disorders • Obsessive-compulsive disorder

KEY POINTS

- Radiosurgery with small-beam collimation at doses higher than 100 Gy to the thalamus can be used to treat tremor.
- There is renewed interest in radiosurgical lesioning of the anterior internal capsule (anterior capsulotomy) in patients with medically refractory obsessive-compulsive disorder.
- Radiosurgery has an expanding role in the management of focal epilepsy disorders such as mesial temporal sclerosis. Research trials are ongoing.

INTRODUCTION

The history of stereotactic radiosurgery begins within the history of functional neurosurgery. When Leksell initially conceived the idea of precise, single-session irradiation of a precisely defined brain target in 1951, he first applied this concept to functional neurosurgery.[1] Radiosurgery was used to obtain closed-skull ablation at a time when either thermal energy or chemical injection was common. Leksell crossfired photon or proton radiation beams to achieve a similar goal. The initial radiosurgical concept was to create a small, precisely defined focal lesion, which was defined by image guidance. The procedure would not completely avoid brain penetration, because contrast encephalography provided the information for identification of the targets. Whereas the ganglionic portion of the trigeminal nerve could be indirectly located using plain radiographs or cisternograms, deep brain targets required air or positive contrast ventriculography. Direct target identification for functional radiosurgery required the later development of computed tomography. The lack of electrophysiologic guidance was controversial, and this remained the greatest argument against the use of radiosurgery for selected disorders. Nevertheless, the current use of radiosurgery as a lesion generator is based on extensive animal studies that defined the dose, volume, and temporal response of the irradiated tissue. The usefulness of radiosurgery has now been compared with microsurgical, percutaneous injection, and electrode-based techniques used for functional neurologic disorders. Current anatomic targets include the trigeminal nerve and sphenopalatine ganglion, the thalamus (for tremor or pain), the anterior internal capsule or cingulum (for

Disclosures: Dr. Lunsford is a consultant for Elekta AB.

[a] Department of Neurosurgery, NYU Langone Medical Center, 530 First Avenue, Suite 8R, New York, NY 10016, USA; [b] Department of Radiation Oncology, University of Pittsburgh Medical Center, Pittsburgh, PA, USA; [c] Department of Neurological Surgery, University of Pittsburgh Medical Center, 200 Lothrop Street, Suite B-400, Pittsburgh, PA 15213, USA
* Corresponding author.
E-mail address: douglas.kondziolka@nyumc.org

behavioral disorders), the hypothalamus (for cancer pain), and the hippocampus or other brain targets (for epilepsy).[2,3]

Leksell first coupled an orthovoltage x-ray tube to his early-generation stereotactic frame, a concept used for trigeminal neuralgia but not for intraparenchymal brain targets.[4] Thus, he began work with physicist Borje Larsson to crossfire proton beams[5] and subsequently used a modified linear accelerator. His decision to build and then use the first Gamma Knife in 1967 reflected his desire for a dedicated, efficient, in-hospital system. As originally designed, the first Gamma Knife collimator helmets created a discoid volume of focal irradiation that could section white matter tracts or brain tissue in a manner similar to an open surgical instrument. Later models of the Gamma Knife allowed the creation of lesions or effects of different volumes, together with precise robotic delivery and efficiency.

Early Development

Before 1978, all uses of radiosurgery remained limited because of the lack of high-resolution, neuroimaging techniques to identify brain lesions or functional brain regions. Angiographic targeting of arteriovenous malformations proved successful, but still was limited by the two-dimensional estimates of complex target volumes, and difficulty with integrating the contributions of multiple isocenters. Functional radiosurgery was performed for a few patients with intractable pain related to malignancy,[6,7] movement disorders,[2] psychiatric dysfunction,[6,8] and trigeminal neuralgia.[4] In the early 1970s, percutaneous retrogasserian glycerol rhizotomy was developed during an observation made during the refinement of the Gamma Knife technique for trigeminal neuralgia. Hakänsson and Leksell attempted to localize the trigeminal nerve within its cistern using glycerol mixed with tantalum powder (as a radiopaque marker) placed before radiosurgery. However, after injection of the glycerol, trigeminal neuralgia pain was relieved.

For intractable pain related to malignancy, radiosurgery was used both for hypophysectomy as well as for medial thalamotomy. Although the procedure was noninvasive, the latency interval for lesion generation and pain relief was 1 major limitation. Steiner and colleagues[7] presented results from an autopsy study after radiosurgery for cancer pain in 1980. Animal experiments using photons and protons proved helpful in determining the ablative dose to be used in patients.[5,9,10] Initial patients who had radiosurgery for tissue ablation received maximum doses of 100 to 250 Gy. At small volumes, doses in excess of 150 Gy provided consistent tissue necrosis in animal models. Many of these first patients had advanced cancer and did not live long enough to provide information on safety. However, the clinical use of such doses proved to be the foundation for later use in tremor management.

Dose Selection

Early animal experiments showed consistent lesion creation at doses at or higher than 150 Gy.[9,10] In patients, pain relief occurred usually within 3 weeks after radiosurgery.[7] In rat experiments at 200 Gy using a single 4-mm isocenter, we found a consistent relationship for lesion generation that substantiated observations from that human study.[11] Doses of 200 Gy were delivered to the rat frontal brain and then the brain was studied at 1, 7, 14, 21, 60, and 90 days after irradiation. At 1 and 7 days, we noted that the brain continued to appear normal. By 14 days, the parenchyma appeared slightly edematous within the target volume. However, by 21 days, a complete circumscribed volume of necrosis was identified within the radiation volume (4 mm diameter). Thus, the clinical observation of pain relief at 21 days noted by Steiner and colleagues was correlated with laboratory findings at the 200-Gy dose.

The ablative radiosurgery lesion appears as a discrete, circumscribed volume of complete parenchymal necrosis with cavitation. Within a 1-mm to 3-mm rim that characterizes the steep fall-off in radiation dose, normalization of the tissue appearance is found. In this zone, blood vessels appear thickened and hyalinized, and often protein extravasation can be identified. Inflammatory changes are noted in this region. Magnetic resonance imaging (MRI) shows all of these features after radiosurgical thalamotomy: a sharply defined, contrast-enhanced rim that defines the low signal lesion (on short repetition time [TR] images) surrounded by a zone of high-signal (on long TR images) brain tissue. Friehs and colleagues[12] collected imaging data from 4 centers that created functional radiosurgery lesions (n = 56). These investigators found that maximum doses in excess of 160 Gy were more likely to produce lesions larger than expected and recommended single 4-mm isocenter lesions at doses lower than 160 Gy. The inflammatory changes can be treated with corticosteroid or other agents should they prove symptomatic in humans.

Studies at the University of Pittsburgh found that in both large-animal and small-animal models, doses at or higher than 100 Gy caused necrosis, but the delay to necrosis was longer.[11,13] To identify the effect of increasing volume, we used an

8-mm collimator in a baboon model and found that half of the animals developed an 8-mm-diameter necrotic lesion at doses as low as 50 Gy.[14] Additional thalamic studies in baboons using 100 Gy and a 4-mm collimator found 3-mm necrotic lesions at 6 months. Dose, volume, and time are the 3 key factors that determine the nature of the functional ablative lesion. Once created, this lesion remains stable over years.[9]

Dose and volume effects are usually, but not always, reliable. The greatest reproducibility is with the smallest targets. When a larger brain target is desirable, the sharp fall-off in dose outside the target becomes less steep with increasing volume. The risk of an adverse radiation effect outside the target volume must be considered, and dose selection is crucial.[15]

Imaging in Functional Surgery

Because physiologic information is excluded from the targeting component of a functional radiosurgery procedure, high-quality, accurate stereotactic neuroimaging must be performed. In addition, the imaging must be of sufficient resolution to identify the target structure but regional anatomy.[16] MRI is the preferred imaging tool for functional radiosurgery.[16–18] Computed tomography can be used with 1-mm to 1.25-mm slice thicknesses in patients with a contraindication to MRI.

The use of fast inversion recovery or other MR sequences with a long relaxation time helps to separate gray and white matter structures. However, the targeting of physiologically abnormal brain regions such as groups of kinesthetic thalamic tremor cells or epileptic foci using imaging alone remains indirect. We believe that with improvements in subcortical imaging using higher field strength magnets, Gamma Knife radiosurgery will play an expanded role in movement disorders. We have not considered that 3-T imaging provided any significant benefit over 1.5-T imaging. In 1 patient, we obtained nonstereotactic 7-T images to evaluate thalamic anatomy. Further studies are pending.

Radiosurgical Thalamotomy

Ventrolateral thalamic surgery for the management of tremor related to Parkinson disease (PD) remains a proven and time-honored concept within functional neurosurgery. Traditionally, this surgery has involved imaging definition of the thalamic target, placement of an electrode into the thalamus, physiologic recording and stimulation at the target site, and creation of a lesion or providing electrical stimulation. Radiosurgical thalamotomy by definition avoids placement of the electrode

and evaluation of the physiologic response. In radiosurgery, imaging definition alone is used to determine lesion placement. Through the use of contrast ventriculography, computed tomographic imaging, and more recently stereotactic MRI, thalamotomy using the Gamma Knife has been performed at centers across the world.[17,19–21] As discussed earlier, the issues of lesion volume and dose selection remain important. Although radiosurgery can abolish tremor, many surgeons believe that although adequate results might be obtained, better results may be possible with deep brain stimulation (DBS). The challenges inherent in choosing the best possible ablative target using imaging alone are significant. Radiosurgical thalamotomy, if performed, should be performed by surgeons experienced in radiofrequency thalamotomy or DBS.

Because of the absence of electrophysiologic information, the inability to stop the lesion during surgery, and the latency to the clinical response, most surgeons use radiosurgery primarily for patients with advanced age or medical disorders, in whom electrode placement would be associated with higher risk. Ohye[20] began to perform radiosurgical thalamotomy contralateral to a previous radiofrequency lesion or to enlarge a previously mapped lesion. Duma and colleagues[17] reported a 5-year experience with 38 thalamotomies using the Gamma Knife and 28-month mean follow-up. Complete tremor abolition was noted in 24%, excellent relief in 26%, good improvement in 29%, and little to no benefit in 21%. The median time to improvement was 2 months, consistent with data from previous animal experiments. They used a dose range of 110 to 165 Gy with better results at higher doses. Such higher doses may exert effects on a larger surrounding tissue volume of kinesthetic tremor cells (outside the sharply defined necrotic volume), which translates into tremor reduction and overcomes any limitations in target selection. Young and colleagues[22] reported that 88% of 27 patients who had radiosurgical thalamotomy for tremor (120–160 Gy) became tremor free or nearly tremor free. Hirato and colleagues[19] also found tremor suppression after GKT in a small patient series. Friehs and colleagues[21] reported an experience of radiosurgical thalamotomy (n = 3) and caudatotomy (n = 10) with clinical improvement in most patients and no morbidity.

Our first report was published in 2008 and focused on essential tremor (ET).[23] Gamma Knife radiosurgery proved to be effective in improving medically refractory ET in a predominantly elderly patient series. We recently evaluated our series of 86 patients with postradiosurgery evaluations who had either ET, PD, or multiple sclerosis.[24] The median follow-up after gamma knife thalamotomy (GKT) was 11.5 months (range 1–152 months). The Fahn-Tolosa-Marin (FTM) clinical tremor rating scale was used to assess preoperative and postoperative tremor, handwriting, and ability to drink from a cup. Benefit was noted at an average of 2 months. Among the 48 treated patients who had ET, the mean preoperative FTM writing score was 2.7 ± 0.8 and mean postoperative writing score was 1.4 ± 1.1 ($P<.00001$). The tremor score was 3.3 ± 0.8 preoperatively and 1.8 ± 1.2 ($P<.00001$) postoperatively. The water score improved from 3.1 ± 0.8 before GKT to 1.7 ± 1.2 ($P<.00001$) at the most recent follow-up. Of those diagnosed with ET, 20 patients (48%) showed either complete resolution or a barely perceivable tremor after GKT.

Among 29 patients with PD who underwent GKT, the mean FTM writing score changed from 2.4 ± 0.6 preoperatively to 1.3 ± 0.9 ($P<.0001$) afterward. The mean tremor score was 3.0 ± 0.8 before GKT and 1.5 ± 1.1 ($P<.0001$) after GKT, and the mean water score was 2.9 ± 0.8 before treatment and 1.5 ± 1.0 ($P<.0001$) after treatment. Results for the 11 patients with multiple sclerosis showed mean writing scores of 3.7 ± 0.5 before GKT and 2.4 ± 0.8 ($P<.003$) after GKT. Mean tremor scores were 3.9 ± 0.3 preoperatively and 2.5 ± 0.9 ($P<.001$) postoperatively. Mean pretreatment FTM drinking scores were 3.9 ± 0.3 and 2.5 ± 1.0 ($P<.003$) at the most recent follow-up. Patients with MS had significantly higher preoperative scores but showed a similar FTM score improvement after GKT: an improvement of 1.3 in writing score, an improvement of 1.4 in tremor score, and an improvement of 1.4 in the drinking score. Two patients experienced temporary contralateral hemiparesis 6 months after GKT, 1 patient experienced dysphagia after 8 months, and 1 patient described a perioral burning sensation with left-sided facial numbness.

The thalamotomy lesion that developed in patients was visible on the first MRI scan (obtained as early as 3 months). MRI imaging was requested 4 months after radiosurgery and was not routinely repeated unless new symptoms developed, because in an early cohort of patients the observed lesions remained stable for 2 years and then decreased in size (**Fig. 1**). The effect was a well-circumscribed contrast-enhanced lesion with central hypointensity. The mean contrast-enhanced short TR MRI lesion diameter was 5 mm. Few patients underwent MRI after 1 year but persistent contrast-enhanced lesions could be seen within years 1 to 2, with regression of enhancement after year 2. The patients who had any complication had onset of symptoms beginning at 6 months after thalamotomy. Imaging performed at that time showed evidence of larger contrast-enhancing lesions as a result of blood-brain barrier disruption with inflammation, and later regression. In a recent multicenter report from Japan, 72 patients with PD and ET were described.[20] The dose was 130 Gy. Of 53 patients who completed 24 months of follow-up, 43 were found to have excellent or good results (81.1%) using formal rating scales.

As noted earlier, the target volume is crucial. Early results with larger target volumes using an 8-mm collimator were reported by Lindquist and colleagues[2] Delayed cerebral edema and regions of radiation necrosis at high doses testified to the volume effects of radiosurgery.[25] Similar problems have been noted using combinations of 4-mm isocenters to construct a cylindrical rather than spherical target volume.[15,22] Nevertheless, the ability to create a small-volume lesion using radiosurgery without invasive placement of an electrode remain attractive considerations.

Radiosurgical Pallidotomy and Subthalamotomy

There was a resurgence in the use of radiofrequency-based stereotactic pallidotomy for patients with advanced PD beginning in 1992. Some investigators then performed Gamma Knife pallidotomy using image guidance alone as an alternative to electrode techniques. Rand and colleagues[26] reported their preliminary results after radiosurgical pallidotomy and noted relief of contralateral rigidity in 4 of 8 patients. No patient in their series sustained a complication. Friedman and colleagues[27] reported on 4 patients after Gamma Knife pallidotomy (180 Gy), with improvement in only 1 patient. These investigators noted variability in lesion volumes on MRI, a finding also documented by others. These lesions were less consistent than thalamic lesions, perhaps related to effects on perforating arteries.[22] At our center, only 1 radiosurgical pallidotomy has been performed. At present, this technique is performed rarely, and DBS remains a more valuable concept for most patients with an array of PD symptoms.[28]

Gamma Knife radiosurgical subthalamotomy has been performed by neurosurgeons Marcus Keep, Bernardo Perez, and Jean Régis with their respective teams (personal communications, 2013). Outcomes in clinical series remain to be published. Presentations at meetings have shown that this procedure can be safe with 4-mm collimation and a dose of 120 Gy. It may be a

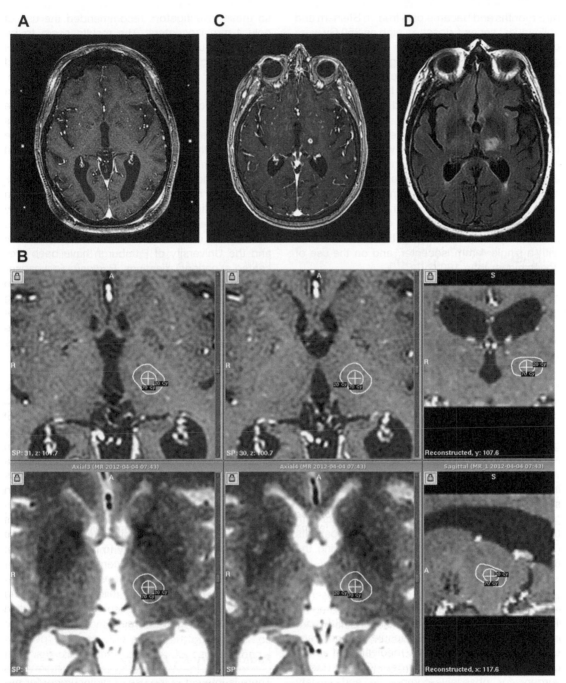

Fig. 1. (*A*) MRI scan at Gamma Knife radiosurgery in an 83-year-old woman with ET. The dose plan is shown (*B*). Significant tremor reduction was noted without side effects. MRI 4 months later shows the contrast-enhanced radiosurgical lesion (*C*) and the peritarget signal change on flair imaging (*D*).

reasonable option in patients not suitable for subthalamic DBS.

Radiosurgery for Pain

The use of radiosurgery as an ablative tool to treat pain has a long history. Too few patients have

been managed to draw any strong conclusions. Since the case report by Leksell[29] in 1968 and the larger series by Steiner and colleagues in 1980,[7] there have been few reports. In Leksell's 2 patients with carcinoma, the centrum medianum target received doses of 250 and 200 Gy.[29] The second patient had bilateral radiosurgery spaced by 2 months and became pain free. In Steinern and colleagues' series,[7] doses as high as 250 Gy were believed unnecessary because of the sharp dose gradient. Young and colleagues[30] performed medial thalamotomy for the treatment of chronic noncancer pain in patients who had failed comprehensive medical, surgical, and behavioral therapies. In 1996, they described that two-thirds of their 41-patient series had at least a 50% reduction in pain intensity estimates, with improvements in physical and social functioning.[3] As might be expected, patients with deafferentation pain responded poorly, but more encouraging results were identified in patients with nociceptive syndromes. These investigators cautioned on the use of larger volumes higher than that obtained with a single 4-mm isocenter, and on the use of doses higher than 160 Gy.

Hayashi and colleagues[31] performed pituitary gland-stalk ablation by Gamma Knife radiosurgery, targeting the border between the pituitary stalk and gland with a maximum dose of 160 Gy using the 8-mm collimator to control cancer pain. They enrolled 9 patients who had bone metastases and pain controlled well by morphine (Karnofsky Performance Status >40) and with no previous radiation therapy. All patients had failed the previous pain treatments except morphine. All patients became pain free within a few days after radiosurgery, which was maintained as long as they lived. No recurrence of pain occurred. In addition, there was no panhypopituitarism and diabetes insipidus in the patients. This strategy of pituitary gland-stalk ablation for pain control also showed a good initial response (87.5%) of 8 patients with thalamic pain syndrome, However, most patients (71.4%) experienced pain recurrence during the 6-month follow-up.[32]

Radiosurgery for Behavioral Disorders

There is renewed interest in radiosurgical lesioning of the anterior internal capsule (anterior capsulotomy) in patients with medically refractory obsessive-compulsive disorder (OCD). Radiosurgery for obsessive-compulsive and anxiety neurosis has been performed for more than 45 years.[6] The first radiosurgical capsulotomy was performed by Leksell in 1953 using 300-kV x-rays.[33] Initially, pneumoencephalography was used for target definition in the placement of bilateral anterior internal capsule lesions. Five of the initial 7 patients had long-term benefit after 7 years of follow-up.[2] Since 1988, an additional 10 patients have been treated at the Karolinska Institute using stereotactic MRI guidance. The initial use of an 8-mm collimator resulted in excessive edema,

so these investigators recommended the use of only 4-mm isocenters. The results seem to be as efficacious as when conventional radiofrequency lesioning is performed.[34] Kihlstrom and colleagues[35] described the stable imaging appearance of radiosurgical lesions 15 to 18 years after capsulotomy. Oval radiosurgical lesions in the anterior internal capsule or cingulate gyrus may affect affective disorders or anxiety neuroses. Recently, Ruck and colleagues[36] reported on long-term follow-up in 25 patients, 16 with an electrode and 9 with Gamma Knife surgery. Response rates did not differ between methods, and these investigators concluded that capsulotomy was effective in reducing OCD symptoms.

A series of patients from Brown University and the University of Pittsburgh have been presented at national meetings. Radiosurgical capsulotomy is performed only after comprehensive psychiatric evaluation and management, leading to a diagnosis of severe OCD, and after failure of nonsurgical approaches. In Pittsburgh, we have performed Gamma Knife surgery on 5 patients with severe, medically intractable OCD (**Fig. 2**). According to our protocol, all patients were evaluated by at least 2 psychiatrists who recommended the capsulotomy procedure. The patient had to request the procedure, and have severe OCD according to the Yale Brown Obsessive Compulsive Scale (YBOCS). Patient ages were 37, 55, and 40 years, and preradiosurgery YBOCS scores were 32/40/39/40, and 39/40. Bilateral lesions were created with 2 4-mm isocenters to create an oval volume in the ventral capsule at the putaminal midpoint. A maximum dose of 140 to 150 Gy was used. There was no morbidity after the procedure and all returned immediately to baseline function. The first 3 patients in our recent report had functional improvements, and reduction in OCD behavior.[37] We believe that this technique should be evaluated further in patients with severe and disabling behavioral disorders.

Radiosurgery for Epilepsy

There is interest in the use of radiosurgery for patients with focal epilepsy. The observation that brain irradiation (via radiation therapy or radiosurgery) could lead to cessation of seizures has spurred several groups to work in this field despite the lack of a consistent approach to defining the target volume. In 1985, Barcia-Salorio and colleagues[38] reported on 6 patients with epilepsy who had low-dose radiosurgery. The epileptic focus was localized by means of conventional scalp electroencephalogram (EEG), subarachnoid electrodes, and depth electrodes. Radiosurgery

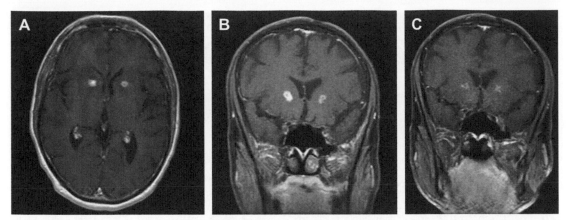

Fig. 2. Bilateral anterior capsulotomies are shown on coronal contrast-enhanced MRI, 1 year after Gamma Knife radiosurgery (140 Gy) in a patient with OCD (*A*, axial; *B*, coronal). Two years after radiosurgery, the degree of contrast enhancement is less (*C*).

(a 10-mm collimator to deliver an estimated dose of 10 Gy) was performed using a cobalt unit coupled to a stereotactic localizer. These investigators hypothesized that this low radiation dose provided a specific effect on epileptic neurons, without inducing tissue necrosis. In 1994, they provided a long-term analysis in a series of 11 patients using a dose range of 10 to 20 Gy.[39] Five patients had complete cessation of seizures, and an additional 5 were improved. Seizures began to decrease gradually after 3 to 12 months after radiosurgery. After this work, Lindquist and colleagues[2] at the Karolinska Institute began to perform epilepsy radiosurgery using advanced localization techniques, which included magnetoencephalography (MEG) to define interictal activity.[40] In some patients, the epileptic dipole activity identified on MEG before radiosurgery later resolved along with seizure cessation. Radiosurgery was evaluated in animal models of epilepsy. We used the kainic acid model of hippocampal epilepsy in the rat, and were able to stop seizures and improve animal behavior.[41,42] Rats were randomized to control or radiosurgery arms (20, 40, 60, or 100 Gy) and then evaluated with serial EEG, behavioral studies, functional MRI, and histology.

More recently, radiosurgery has been of value in patients with gelastic or generalized seizures related to hypothalamic hamartomas.[43] A larger indication may rest with the use of epilepsy to create an amygdalohippocampal lesion for patients with mesial temporal sclerosis as proposed by Régis and colleagues.[44,45] In 1993, Régis and associates in Marseille performed selective amygdalohippocampal radiosurgery for mesial temporal lobe epilepsy. Gamma Knife radiosurgery was used to create a conformal volume of radiation for the amygdala and hippocampus. This approximate 7-mL volume represented the largest functional target irradiated to that time. They delivered a margin dose of 25 Gy to the 50% isodose line, a dose that later caused target necrosis. The first patient became seizure free immediately and the second after a latency of almost 1 year. Serial MRI scans showed target contrast enhancement that corresponded to the 50% isodose line. Patients managed at their center have been part of a multidisciplinary prospective evaluation and treatment protocol. A recently published longer-term evaluation with 8-year mean follow-up (margin dose of 24 Gy), found that 9 of 16 patients were seizure free.[46] The 2010 review by Régis and colleagues[44] on their experience with functional radiosurgery is excellent.

The first prospective multicenter clinical trial in the United States was recently completed.[47] This study with 3-year outcomes evaluated effects on epilepsy, cognition, and neurologic function. Seizure control was higher at 48 Gy compared with 40 Gy, and similar to what is reported after hippocampectomy. Neuropsychological testing reported that radiosurgery was safe. However, several important questions remain to be addressed regarding the role of radiosurgery for mesial temporal sclerosis-related epilepsy. The optimal target may include both amygdala and hippocampus, but the total target volume remains debated (**Fig. 3**). Target volume helps to determine dose selection, including the dose received by regional structures such as the brainstem or optic tract. Investigators need to determine whether the balance between seizure response and morbidity is acceptable, particularly compared with surgical resection. For these reasons, a randomized trial comparing radiosurgery with resection was begun under the leadership of

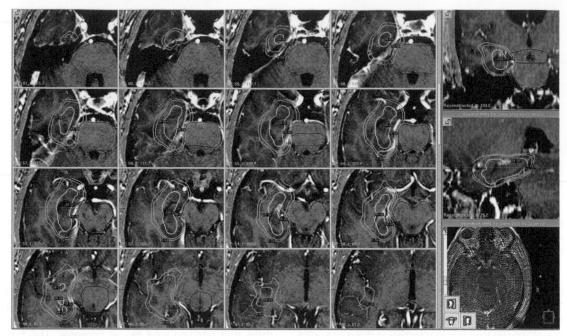

Fig. 3. Gamma Knife radiosurgery plan in a 56-year-old man with mesial temporal sclerosis.

Dr Nicholas Barbaro (Indiana University) and Dr Mark Quigg (University of Virginia). Entitled the Radiosurgery or Surgery for Epilepsy (ROSE) trial, the study is under way at centers in several countries.

Current issues that remain important for epilepsy radiosurgery include dose selection (necrotizing vs nonnecrotizing), localization methods for non-lesional epilepsy, the target volume necessary for irradiation, and the expected short-term and long-term outcomes. Some groups have used low doses (10–20 Gy) when few if any histologic changes would be expected. Others have used doses as high as 100 Gy, which cause target necrosis and regional brain edema.[48] From recent trials, a common amygdalohippocampal radiosurgery maximum dose to a volume less than 7.5 mL is 40 to 50 Gy.

Functional Imaging and Radiosurgery

Improvements in functional imaging will affect radiosurgery. Functional MRI to localize cortical function before radiosurgery has been evaluated in pilot studies. Localization of motor function and speech areas surrounding arteriovenous malformations and brain tumors before radiosurgery has assisted dose planning.[49] This information can be used to restrict the radiosurgery dose away from functional areas. Advancements in functional imaging may improve the localization of epileptic foci, and perhaps even regions of

excitation in the basal ganglia. Magnetoencephalography is an exciting tool to identify functional activation. An ability to identify hyperactivity in deep brain structures would be valuable. High-definition fiber tracking using diffusion tensor imaging is being evaluated in patients with movement and other neurodegenerative disorders. With further improvements in neuroimaging and noninvasive physiologic studies, the future will see a significant linkage between functional brain disorders and stereotactic radiosurgery.

REFERENCES

1. Leksell L. The stereotaxic method and radiosurgery of the brain. Acta Chir Scand 1951;102: 316–9.
2. Lindquist C, Kihlstrom L, Hellstrand DE. Functional neurosurgery–a future for the Gamma Knife? Stereotact Funct Neurosurg 1991;57:72–81.
3. Young RF, Vermeulen S, Posewitz A, et al. Functional neurosurgery with the Leksell Gamma knife. Stereotact Funct Neurosurg 1996;66:19–23.
4. Leksell L. Stereotaxic radiosurgery in trigeminal neuralgia. Acta Chir Scand 1971;137:311–4.
5. Larsson B, Leksell L, Rexed B, et al. The high-energy proton beam as a neurosurgical tool. Nature 1958;182:1222–3.
6. Leksell L, Backlund EO. Stereotactic gammacapsulotomy. In: Hitchcock ER, Ballantine HT, Meyerson BA, editors. Modern concepts in psychiatric surgery. Amsterdam: Elsevier; 1979. p. 213–6.

7. Steiner L, Forster D, Leksell L, et al. Gammathalamotomy in intractable pain. Acta Neurochir 1980; 52:173–84.

8. Rylander G. Stereotactic radiosurgery in anxiety and obsessive-compulsive states: psychiatric aspects. In: Hitchcock ER, Ballantine HT, Meyerson BA, editors. Modern concepts in psychiatric surgery. Amsterdam: Elsevier; 1979. p. 235–40.

9. Andersson B, Larsson B, Leksell L, et al. Histopathology of late local radiolesions in the goat brain. Acta Radiol Ther Phys Biol 1970;9:385–94.

10. Rexed B, Mair W, Sourander P, et al. Effect of high energy protons on the brain of the rabbit. Acta Radiol Ther Phys Biol 1960;53:289–99.

11. Kondziolka D, Lunsford LD, Claassen D, et al. Radiobiology of radiosurgery. Part I: the normal rat brain model. Neurosurgery 1992;31:271–9.

12. Friehs G, Noren G, Ohye C, et al. Lesion size following Gamma Knife treatment for functional disorders. Stereotact Funct Neurosurg 1996;66(Suppl 1): 320–8.

13. Kondziolka D, Linskey ME, Lunsford LD. Animal models in radiosurgery. In: Alexander E, Loeffler JS, Lunsford LD, editors. Stereotactic radiosurgery. New York: McGraw-Hill; 1993. p. 51–64.

14. Lunsford LD, Altschuler EM, Flickinger JC, et al. In vivo biological effects of stereotactic radiosurgery: a primate model. Neurosurgery 1990;27: 373–82.

15. Kihlstrom L, Guo WY, Lindquist C, et al. Radiobiology of radiosurgery for refractory anxiety disorders. Neurosurgery 1995;36:294–302.

16. Kondziolka D, Dempsey PK, Lunsford LD, et al. A comparison between magnetic resonance imaging and computed tomography for stereotactic coordinate determination. Neurosurgery 1992;30:402–7.

17. Duma C, Jacques D, Kopyov O, et al. Gamma Knife radiosurgery for thalamotomy in Parkinsonian tremor: a five-year experience. Neurosurg Focus 1997;2(3):E14.

18. Kondziolka D, Lunsford LD, Flickinger JC, et al. Stereotactic radiosurgery for trigeminal neuralgia: a multi-institution study using the gamma unit. J Neurosurg 1996;84:940–5.

19. Hirato M, Ohye C, Shibazaki T, et al. Gamma Knife thalamotomy for the treatment of functional disorders. Stereotact Funct Neurosurg 1995;64(Suppl 1): 164–71.

20. Ohye C, Higuchi Y, Shibazaki T, et al. Gamma Knife thalamotomy for Parkinson disease and essential tremor: a prospective multicenter study. Neurosurgery 2012;70:526–36.

21. Friehs G, Ojakangas CL, Pachatz P, et al. Thalamotomy and caudatomy with the Gamma Knife as a treatment for Parkinsonism with a comment on lesion sizes. Stereotact Funct Neurosurg 1995;64(Suppl 1): 209–21.

22. Young RF, Shumway-Cook A, Vermeulen S, et al. Gamma Knife radiosurgery as a lesioning technique in movement disorder surgery. Neurosurg Focus 1997;2(3):e11.

23. Kondziolka D, Ong J, Lee JY, et al. Gamma Knife thalamotomy for essential tremor. J Neurosurg 2008;108:111–7.

24. Kooshkabadi A, Lunsford LD, Tonetti D, et al. Gamma Knife thalamotomy for tremor in the MRI era. J Neurosurg 2013;118(4):713–8.

25. Leksell L, Herner T, Leksell D, et al. Visualization of stereotactic radiolesions by nuclear magnetic resonance. J Neurol Neurosurg Psychiatry 1985; 48:19–20.

26. Rand RW, Jacques DB, Melbye RW, et al. Gamma Knife thalamotomy and pallidotomy in patients with movement disorders: preliminary results. Stereotact Funct Neurosurg 1993;61(Suppl 1):65–92.

27. Friedman J, Epstein M, Sanes J, et al. Gamma knife pallidotomy in advanced Parkinson's disease. Ann Neurol 1996;39:535–8.

28. Kwon Y, Whang CJ. Stereotactic Gamma Knife radiosurgery for the treatment of dystonia. Stereotact Funct Neurosurg 1995;64(Suppl 1):222–7.

29. Leksell L. Cerebral radiosurgery I. Gammathalamotomy in two cases of intractable pain. Acta Chir Scand 1968;134:585–95.

30. Young RF, Jacques DB, Rand RW, et al. Medial thalamotomy with the Leksell Gamma Knife for treatment of chronic pain. Acta Neurochir 1994;62: 105–10.

31. Hayashi M, Taira T, Chernov M, et al. Gamma Knife surgery for cancer pain-pituitary gland-stalk ablation: a multicenter prospective protocol since 2002. J Neurosurg 2002;97:433–7.

32. Hayashi M, Taira T, Chernov M, et al. Role of pituitary radiosurgery for the management of intractable pain and potential future applications. Stereotact Funct Neurosurg 2003;81:75–83.

33. Leksell L, Herner T, Liden K. Stereotaxic radiosurgery of the brain. Report of a case. Kungl Fysiogr Sallsk Lund Forhandl 1995;25:1–10.

34. Alexander E, Lindquist C. Special indications: radiosurgery for functional neurosurgery and epilepsy. In: Alexander E, Loeffler JS, Lunsford LD, editors. Stereotactic radiosurgery. New York: McGraw-Hill; 1993. p. 221–5.

35. Kihlstrom L, Hindmarsh T, Lax I, et al. Radiosurgical lesions in the normal human brain 17 years after Gamma Knife capsulotomy. Neurosurgery 1997;41: 396–402.

36. Ruck C, Karlsson A, Steele JD, et al. Capsulotomy for obsessive-compulsive disorder. Long-term follow-up of 25 patients. Arch Gen Psychiatry 2008;65:914–22.

37. Kondziolka D, Hudak R, Flickinger JC. Results following gamma knife radiosurgical anterior

capsulotomies for obsessive compulsive disorder. Neurosurgery 2011;68:28–33.

38. Salorio JL, Roldan P, Hernandez G, et al. Radiosurgical treatment of epilepsy. Stereotact Funct Neurosurg 1985;48(1–6):400–3.

39. Barcia-Salorio JL, Barcia JA, Hernandez G, et al. Radiosurgery of epilepsy. Long-term results. Acta Neurochir 1994;62(Suppl):111.

40. Hellstrand DE, Abraham-Fuchs K, Jernberg B, et al. MEG localization of interictal epileptic focal activity and concomitant stereotactic radiosurgery. A non-invasive approach for patient with focal epilepsy. Physiol Meas 1993;14:131–6.

41. Maesawa S, Kondziolka D, Dixon E, et al. Subnecrotic stereotactic radiosurgery controlling epilepsy produced by kainic acid injection in rats. J Neurosurg 2000;93:1033–40.

42. Mori Y, Kondziolka D, Balzer J, et al. Effects of stereotactic radiosurgery on an animal model of hippocampal epilepsy. Neurosurgery 2000;46:157–68.

43. Mathieu D, Kondziolka D, Niranjan A, et al. Gamma knife radiosurgery for epilepsy caused by hypothalamic hamartomas. Stereotact Funct Neurosurg 2006;84:82–7.

44. Régis J, Carron R, Park M. Is radiosurgery a neuromodulation therapy? A 2009 Fabrikant Award Lecture. J Neurooncol 2010;98:155–62.

45. Régis J, Rey M, Bartolomei F, et al. Gamma knife surgery in mesial temporal lobe epilepsy: a prospective multicenter study. Epilepsia 2004;45:504–15.

46. Bartolomei F, Hayashi M, Tamura M, et al. Long-term efficacy of gamma knife radiosurgery in mesial temporal lobe epilepsy. Neurology 2008;70:1658–63.

47. Barbaro NN, Quigg M, Broshek D, et al. A multicenter, prospective pilot study of Gamma Knife radiosurgery for mesial temporal lobe epilepsy: seizure response, adverse events, and verbal memory. Ann Neurol 2009;65:167–75.

48. Whang CJ, Kim CJ. Short-term follow-up of stereotactic Gamma Knife radiosurgery in epilepsy. Stereotact Funct Neurosurg 1995;64(Suppl 1):202–8.

49. Witt TC, Kondziolka D, Baumann S, et al. Pre-operative cortical localization with functional MRI for use in stereotactic radiosurgery. Stereotact Funct Neurosurg 1996;66:24–9.

Index

Note: Page numbers of article titles are in **boldface** type.

Neurosurg Clin N Am 24 (2013) 633–636
http://dx.doi.org/10.1016/S1042-3680(13)00072-7
1042-3680/13/$ – see front matter © 2013 Elsevier Inc. All rights reserved.

United States Postal Service

Statement of Ownership, Management, and Circulation
(All Periodicals Publications Except Requestor Publications)

1. Publication Title	2. Publication Number	3. Filing Date
Neurosurgery Clinics of North America	0 1 3 - 1 2 4	9/14/13

4. Issue Frequency	5. Number of Issues Published Annually	6. Annual Subscription Price
Jan, Apr, Jul, Oct	4	$360.00

7. Complete Mailing Address of Known Office of Publication (*Not printer*) (*Street, city, county, state, and ZIP+4®*)

Elsevier Inc.
360 Park Avenue South
New York, NY 10010-1710

Contact Person: Stephen R. Bushing

Telephone (Include area code): 215-239-3688

8. Complete Mailing Address of Headquarters or General Business Office of Publisher (*Not printer*)

Elsevier Inc., 360 Park Avenue South, New York, NY 10010-1710

9. Full Names and Complete Mailing Addresses of Publisher, Editor, and Managing Editor (*Do not leave blank*)

Publisher (*Name and complete mailing address*)

Linda Belfus, Elsevier, Inc., 1600 John F. Kennedy Blvd. Suite 1800, Philadelphia, PA 19103-2899

Editor (*Name and complete mailing address*)

Jessica McCool, Elsevier, Inc., 1600 John F. Kennedy Blvd. Suite 1800, Philadelphia, PA 19103-2899

Managing Editor (*Name and complete mailing address*)

Barbara Cohen-Kligerman, Elsevier, Inc., 1600 John F. Kennedy Blvd. Suite 1800, Philadelphia, PA 19103-2899

10. Owner (*Do not leave blank. If the publication is owned by a corporation, give the name and address of the corporation immediately followed by the names and addresses of all stockholders owning or holding 1 percent or more of the total amount of stock. If not owned by a corporation, give the names and addresses of the individual owners. If owned by a partnership or other unincorporated firm, give its name and address as well as those of each individual owner. If the publication is published by a nonprofit organization, give its name and address.*)

Full Name	Complete Mailing Address
Wholly owned subsidiary of	1600 John F. Kennedy Blvd., Ste. 1800
Reed/Elsevier, US holdings	Philadelphia, PA 19103-2899

11. Known Bondholders, Mortgagees, and Other Security Holders Owning or Holding 1 Percent or More of Total Amount of Bonds, Mortgages, or Other Securities. If none, check box ☑ None

Full Name	Complete Mailing Address
N/A	

12. Tax Status (*For completion by nonprofit organizations authorized to mail at nonprofit rates*) (*Check one*)
The purpose, function, and nonprofit status of this organization and the exempt status for federal income tax purposes:
☐ Has Not Changed During Preceding 12 Months
☐ Has Changed During Preceding 12 Months (*Publisher must submit explanation of change with this statement*)

PS Form 3526, September 2007 (Page 1 of 3 (Instructions Page 3)) PSN 7530-01-000-9931 PRIVACY NOTICE: See our Privacy policy in www.usps.com

---

13. Publication Title	14. Issue Date for Circulation Data Below
Neurosurgery Clinics of North America	July 2013

15. Extent and Nature of Circulation			Average No. Copies Each Issue During Preceding 12 Months	No. Copies of Single Issue Published Nearest to Filing Date
a. Total Number of Copies (*Net press run*)			606	540
b. Paid Circulation (By Mail and Outside the Mail)	(1)	Mailed Outside-County Paid Subscriptions Stated on PS Form 3541. (*Include paid distribution above nominal rate, advertiser's proof copies, and exchange copies*)	231	199
	(2)	Mailed In-County Paid Subscriptions Stated on PS Form 3541 (*Include paid distribution above nominal rate, advertiser's proof copies, and exchange copies*)		
	(3)	Paid Distribution Outside the Mails Including Sales Through Dealers and Carriers, Street Vendors, Counter Sales, and Other Paid Distribution Outside USPS®	132	138
	(4)	Paid Distribution by Other Classes Mailed Through the USPS (e.g. First-Class Mail®)		
c. Total Paid Distribution (*Sum of 15b (1), (2), (3), and (4)*) ▲			363	337
d. Free or Nominal Rate Distribution (By Mail and Outside the Mail)	(1)	Free or Nominal Rate Outside-County Copies Included on PS Form 3541	51	46
	(2)	Free or Nominal Rate In-County Copies Included on PS Form 3541		
	(3)	Free or Nominal Rate Copies Mailed at Other Classes Through the USPS (e.g. First-Class Mail)		
	(4)	Free or Nominal Rate Distribution Outside the Mail (Carriers or other means)		
e. Total Free or Nominal Rate Distribution (Sum of 15d (1), (2), (3) and (4)) ▲			51	46
f. Total Distribution (Sum of 15c and 15e) ▲			414	383
g. Copies not Distributed (See instructions to publishers #4 (page #3)) ▲			192	157
h. Total (Sum of 15f and g) ▲			606	540
i. Percent Paid (15c divided by 15f times 100) ▲			87.68%	87.99%

16. Publication of Statement of Ownership

☐ If the publication is a general publication, publication of this statement is required. Will be printed in the **October 2013** issue of this publication. ☐ Publication not required

17. Signature and Title of Editor, Publisher, Business Manager, or Owner

Stephen R. Bushing Date: September 14, 2013

Stephen R. Bushing – Inventory Distribution Coordinator

I certify that all information furnished on this form is true and complete. I understand that anyone who furnishes false or misleading information on this form or who omits material or information requested on the form may be subject to criminal sanctions (including fines and imprisonment) and/or civil sanctions (including civil penalties).

PS Form 3526, September 2007 (Page 2 of 3)

Moving?

Make sure your subscription moves with you!

To notify us of your new address, find your **Clinics Account Number** (located on your mailing label above your name), and contact customer service at:

Email: journalscustomerservice-usa@elsevier.com

800-654-2452 (subscribers in the U.S. & Canada)
314-447-8871 (subscribers outside of the U.S. & Canada)

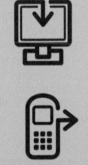

Fax number: 314-447-8029

**Elsevier Health Sciences Division
Subscription Customer Service
3251 Riverport Lane
Maryland Heights, MO 63043**

*To ensure uninterrupted delivery of your subscription, please notify us at least 4 weeks in advance of move.

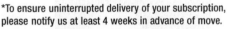

Printed and bound by CPI Group (UK) Ltd, Croydon, CR0 4YY

03/10/2024

01040370-0016